Donald School Textbook of
# DIABETIC PREGNANCY AND ULTRASOUND

Donald School Textbook of
# DIABETIC PREGNANCY AND ULTRASOUND

*Editors*

**Badreldeen Ahmed** FRCOG MD (Newcastle UponTyne) MBCHB MFFP CCST
Professor of Obstetrics
Weill Cornell Medical College, Doha
Director of Feto Maternal Centre
Doha, Qatar

**Asim Kurjak** MD PhD
Professor of Obstetrics and Gynecology
Medical School University of Zagreb
Zagreb, Croatia

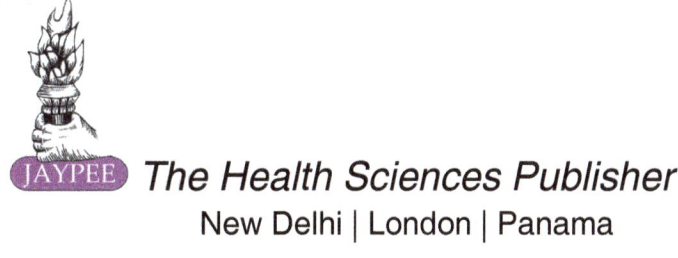

JAYPEE *The Health Sciences Publisher*
New Delhi | London | Panama

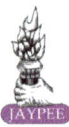 **Jaypee Brothers Medical Publishers (P) Ltd**

**Headquarters**
Jaypee Brothers Medical Publishers (P) Ltd.
4838/24, Ansari Road, Daryaganj
New Delhi 110 002, India
Phone: +91-11-43574357
Fax: +91-11-43574314
E-mail: jaypee@jaypeebrothers.com

**Overseas Offices**

JP Medical Ltd.
83, Victoria Street, London
SW1H 0HW (UK)
Phone: +44-20 3170 8910
Fax: +44(0)20 3008 6180
E-mail: info@jpmedpub.com

Jaypee-Highlights Medical Publishers Inc
City of Knowledge, Bld. 235, 2nd Floor, Clayton
Panama City, Panama
Phone: +1 507-301-0496
Fax: +1 507-301-0499
Email: cservice@jphmedical.com

Jaypee Brothers Medical Publishers (P) Ltd.
17/1-B, Babar Road, Block-B, Shyamoli
Mohammadpur, Dhaka-1207
Bangladesh
Mobile: +08801912003485
E-mail: jaypeedhaka@gmail.com

Jaypee Brothers Medical Publishers (P) Ltd.
Bhotahity, Kathmandu, Nepal
Phone: +977-9741283608
E-mail: kathmandu@jaypeebrothers.com

Website: www.jaypeebrothers.com
Website: www.jaypeedigital.com

Inquiries for bulk sales may be solicited at: jaypee@jaypeebrothers.com

*Donald School Textbook of Diabetic Pregnancy and Ultrasound*

*First Edition:* 2018

ISBN: 978-93-5270-196-4

*Printed at:*

## Dedication

*I dedicate this book to my wife Mandy and my son Kareem,
for their continuous and unconditioned support*

**—Badreldeen Ahmed**

*This book is dedicated to my grandchildren: Dea, Lina, Lara, Din and Dal*

**—Asim Kurjak**

# Contributors

**Badreldeen Ahmed** FRCOG MD (Newcastle UponTyne) MBCHB MFFP CCST
Professor of Obstetrics
Weill Cornell Medical College, Doha
Director of Feto Maternal Centre
Doha, Qatar

**Olus Api** MD
Professor of Obstetrics and Gynecology
Department of Perinatology
Medipol University School of Medicine
Istanbul, Turkey

**Hisham Arab** MD FRCSC FACOG
Senior Consultant Gynecologist
Dr Arab Medical Center
Jeddah, Saudi Arabia

**Frank A Chervenak** MD
Given Foundation
Professor and Chairman
Department of Obstetrics and Gynecology
Weill Cornell Medicine
New York, USA

**Sertac Esin** MD
Associate Professor
Department of Perinatology
Başkent University School of Medicine
Ankara, Turkey

**Miroslava Gojnic** MD PhD
Professor
School of Medicine, University of Belgrade
Clinic for Gynecology and Obstetrics
Clinical Center of Serbia
Belgrade, Serbia

**Farhat Gothey** Pg Dip in Clinical Ultrasound
Sonographer/System Administrator
Women's Clinical Management Group
Sidra Medicine
Doha, Qatar

**Karim D Kalache** MD PhD
Professor of Obstetrics and Gynecology
Weill Cornell Medical College, Qatar
Division Chief, Maternal-Fetal Medicine
Women's Clinical Management Group
Sidra Medicine
Doha, Qatar

**Daniel Kamil** MD
Associate Professor of Obstetrics and Gynecology
Weill Cornell Medical College, Qatar
Senior Attending Physician
Women's Clinical Management Group
Sidra Medicine
Doha, Qatar

**Justin Konje**
FWACS FMCOG (Nig) FRCOG MD MBA LLB PgCert Med Ed
Executive Chair
Women's Services Clinical Management Group
Sidra Medical and Research Center
Doha, Qatar

**Asim Kurjak** MD PhD
Professor of Obstetrics and Gynecology
Medical School University of Zagreb
Zagreb, Croatia

**Sonal Panchal** MD
Consultant Sonography Specialist
Department of Ultrasound
Dr Nagori's Institute for Infertility and IVF
Ahmedabad, Gujarat, India

**Igor V Pantic** MD PhD
Associate Professor
School of Medicine
University of Belgrade
Institute of Medical Physiology
Belgrade, Serbia

**Milan Perovic** MD PhD
Consultant
Clinic for Gynecology and Obstetrics
"Narodni front"
Faculty of Health, Legal and Business Studies
Singidunum University
Belgrade, Serbia

**Cihat Sen** MD
Professor and Chairman
Department of Perinatology
Cerrahpasa Medical School
Istanbul University
Istanbul, Turkey

**Milan Stanojevic** MD PhD
Head of Neonatology
Department of Obstetrics and Gynecology
Medical School University of Zagreb
Neonatal Unit, University Hospital Sveti Duh
Zagreb, Croatia

**Alexander Weichert** MD
Senior Consultant Obstetrician and Gynecologist
Charité University Hospital
Berlin, Germany

**Murat Yayla** MD
Professor of Obstetrics and Gynecology
Consultant on Perinatology
Acıbadem International Hospital
Istanbul, Turkey

# Acknowledgments

We are thankful to Shri Jitendar P Vij (Group Chairman), Mr Ankit Vij (Group President), Ms Chetna Malhotra Vohra (Associate Director–Content Strategy), and Ms Angima Shree (Development Editor) of Jaypee Brothers Medical Publishers, New Delhi, India, for giving us a go-ahead at the very beginning and helping me in every way possible to bring out this book.

# Contents

# Introduction

The profession of perinatal medicine has made great strides in the management of diabetes in pregnancy as manifested by the greatly improved outcomes that have been achieved during the past generation. The *Donald School Textbook of Diabetic Pregnancy* presents an important overview of these advances in a form that the practicing clinician can provide state-of-the-art care for his/her patients. Cihat Sen and his colleagues present the evolving topic of the diagnosis of diabetes in pregnancy as well as an overview of the general aspects of this protean disease. Baldredeen Ahmed and Justin Konje present an overview of the invaluable role of ultrasound in diabetes management while Asim Kurjak and Sonal Panchal present the latest information on the exciting area of fetal behavior evaluation in pregnancy. Karim Kalache and colleagues present the newest developments in ultrasound diagnosis of anomalies in the diabetic pregnancy. The offspring of the diabetic mother is excellently discussed by Milan Stanojevic and Miroslava Gojnic and colleagues. Lastly and importantly, Hisham Arab presents the linkage between diabetes and obesity in pregnancy and beyond.

All clinicians who care for maternal, fetal, and neonatal patients would benefit from this important textbook. It will well-written and well-illustrated and a pleasure to learn from.

**Frank A Chervenak** MD
Given Foundation Professor and Chairman
Department of Obstetrics and Gynecology
Weill Cornell Medicine
New York, USA

# Chapter 1

# Diabetes in Pregnancy: Diagnosis and Treatment

*Cihat Sen, Murat Yayla, Olus Api*

## INTRODUCTION

Gestational diabetes (GD) that is the one of most common medical complications of pregnancy is the dysfunction of glucose metabolism which develops in the second half of pregnancy and disappears when pregnancy ends.[1] Dysfunction of glucose metabolism may have various levels. While diet is sufficient generally, some may need insulin.

Pregestational diabetic and diabetes noticed for the first time during the pregnancy were distinguished from the diabetes cases developing during pregnancy, and two different definitions were set as "gestational diabetes" and "overt diabetes" according to the common definition made by The International Association of Diabetes and Pregnancy Study Group (IADSPG), The World Health Organization (WHO), and The American Diabetes Association (ADA).[2-4] In this case, "gestational diabetes" defines the change which really appears during pregnancy and is diagnosed at the second half of pregnancy by tests and developing in the presence of "pancreas which cannot deal with the diabetogenic changes" of pregnancy.[5] The pregnancy itself is the condition of "physiological insulin resistance". "Overt diabetes" defines the diabetes cases which have the metabolic processes at the early periods of pregnancy almost same with nongestational condition and identified even in the first trimester where insulin resistance is not clear yet. The cases which do not meet "overt diabetes" criteria in the tests performed during gestational period but not found to have a normal carbohydrate metabolism, either, are diagnosed as "gestational diabetes" and their follow-up and treatment are carried out accordingly.

## PREVALENCE

The prevalence of GD is about 3–25% of pregnant women.[6] The main reason for different GD incidence rates among the population investigated is the difference in the incidence rate of type 2 diabetes mellitus (DM) in the society.[7] Also, maternal obesity increasing at young ages, decreased physical activity, increased consumption of convenience food, and advanced maternal age and race are other factors which have impact on prevalence.[7] At the same time, the differences in GD screening models, the threshold values used, and diagnostic criteria create differences in GD prevalence. However, even though different methods and diagnostic criteria are used, it is definite that the prevalence of type 2 DM and also GD has increased in time highly, especially within last 20 years.[5,8]

## PATHOPHYSIOLOGY AND RISK FACTORS

Endocrine and metabolic changes in pregnancy occur right after conception. The main purpose of these changes occurring in maternal metabolism is to provide sufficient nutrient and fuel to fetus.[9] Particularly in the last trimester where fetal growth is the fastest and therefore fetal nutrition need is the highest, the changes in maternal carbohydrate and lipid metabolism become more distinct. During the pregnancy, plasma levels of lipolytic hormones increase and generally maternal fat use elevates, "glucose" is for the use of fetus basically.

Maternal insulin resistance begins at second trimester with the effect of metabolic and hormonal changes and becomes distinctive at third trimester. In this way, insulin resistance increases much more with the increase of the levels of human placental lactogen, human placental growth hormone, estrogen, progesterone, cortisol, prolactin, somatostatin, and probably tumor necrosis factor-alpha (TNF-$\alpha$) that have diabetogenic effects. All these changes reach their peak level approximately at the 30 weeks of gestation. Insulin resistance which develops as a result of normal physiological changes during pregnancy is required for sufficient nutrition and growth of fetus.[9] Since maternal pancreas cannot deal with this situation when increased insulin resistance is encountered, these physiological changes result in GD which is a pathological condition.[5] In fact, pathophysiological mechanisms developing in the formation of GD show similarities substantially with type 2 DM. In both cases, a substantial increase occurs in the insulin resistance as the week of gestation advances and insulin response is not sufficient.

Risk factors for GD are defined and were asserted to perform glucose screening or diagnostic tests in pregnant women having these risk factors. Type 2 DM history in the family (especially in first degree relatives) is related to GD.[10] Also history of GD in previous pregnancy is a risk factor.[11] Another risk factor is obesity [body mass index (BMI) ≥30 kg/m²].[10-12] It is remarkable that 60–80% of GD cases are obese. Also, GD risk increases with BMI.[11] Cardiometabolic risk factors such as pregestational hypertension and borderline high blood pressure values were also associated with increased GD risk.[12] Obesity is associated with inflammatory changes. There is an increase in inflammatory cytokines, especially in the levels of TNF-$\alpha$, interleukin-6, nuclear factor-κB (NFκB), plasminogen activator inhibitor-1 and C-reactive protein.[13] Glucose levels chronically increased with obesity cause the modification of building blocks such as nucleic acids and proteins into advanced glycation end products (AGE). The accumulation of AGE which is fast and higher than physiological levels causes permanent damages in the tissues. Today, AGE formation is held responsible in the physiopathology of many diseases in diabetes cases including neurodegenerative diseases, metabolic syndrome, and vasculopathy.[14] As a respond to AGE formation, a series of inflammatory response is initiated with NFκB pathway, and the tissue damage created with the activation of T-cells and the release of inflammatory cytokines in particular results with vasculopathy and fibrosis.[15,16] Therefore, the development of complications such as myocardial infarction, atherosclerosis, stroke, etc. is not a surprise in obesity and DM patients.[16] The same mechanism may explain the appearance of vascular complications basically such as insufficient placentation, preeclampsia, IUGR, sudden infant death under poor conditions caused by chronic hyperglycemia as well as obesity during pregnancy.

In the diabetes prevalence studies performed in Turkey, DM prevalence was found as 13.7% according to the results of TURDEP-II performed with the participation of 26,000 individuals who were 20 years old and above in 2010.[17] Almost half of the cases in DM group consist of newly diagnosed cases. Diabetes prevalence varies according to the regions in Turkey. While Northern Anatolia Region has the lowest prevalence rate (14.5%), Eastern Anatolia Region has the highest prevalence rate (18.2%). Eastern Anatolia Region was found to be the region with the lowest awareness for diabetes as well as the region having the highest prevalence rate.[17] Compared to TURDEP-I[18] study performed in 1998, the results found by TURDEP-II prevalence study showed that the diabetes prevalence rate increased for 90% and obesity for 44% in Turkey.[17] Another issue revealed by TURDEP-II study is that diabetes prevalence rate increased significantly in those who are in reproductive period.[17]

Considering the worldwide diabetes prevalence is about 8.4%.[19] In the light of these data, our country is among the regions with the highest prevalence according to comparative worldwide diabetes prevalence studies. It is known that GD prevalence is high among those originated from South Asia, black Caribbean, and Middle East.

When planning GD screening program, the characteristics of the population under investigation are also important. For instance, only 10% of the population in the USA is evaluated within low risk group. Therefore, it is wise to perform tests on every pregnant woman instead of carrying out a risk-oriented screening in the USA.[20] Besides, considering the risk factors mentioned earlier, there are few pregnant women left. Hence, it does not seem logical to perform screening based on risk factors.

## Why Screening and Identifying Important?

Clinically identifying GD is significant basically for preventing gestational complications, improving fetal and neonatal outcomes, and to prevent its long-term effects on next generations. While some of the complications developing associated with GD appear in the early period, some of them are seen in the long-term. Preterm labor, macrosomia, birth trauma, and sudden infant death can be listed among the fetal complications associated with GD.[21-23] Among the early period complications in the newborns of GD mothers, there are polycythemia, hyperviscosity, hypoglycemia, hypocalcemia, hyperbilirubinemia, and respiratory distress syndrome (RDS).[24,25] Among the long-term complications, obesity, metabolic syndrome, type 2 DM and increase in hyperactivity prevalence were found in the infants of GD mothers.[26,27] Preeclampsia risk, increased operative labor risk, and polyhydramnios can be listed among the maternal risks.[28,29] Also, the risk for type 2 DM, metabolic syndrome, and coronary artery disease increased in the long-term in GD mothers.[30,31]

Identifying GD in the early period decreases preeclampsia risk for 40% and macrosomic infant risk for 50%. Additionally, shoulder dystocia and brachial plexus palsy risks decrease for 60%. Early detection of GD also decreases stillbirth risk.[32]

## FREQUENT OBSTETRIC AND PERINATAL PROBLEMS IN GESTATIONAL DIABETES

It is known that the presence of chronic hyperglycemia ongoing especially in the last 4–6 weeks of gestation is associated with sudden fetal death associated with possible acidosis even in normal fetuses anatomically.[33,34] Even in GD cases with well-controlled metabolism, fetal macrosomia, neonatal hypoglycemia, polycythemia, and jaundice risks increased although there is no increase in perinatal mortality.[21] Also, cesarean section is recommended when estimated fetal weight is more than or equal to 4,500 g.[1]

## Macrosomia

It is the most common complication seen in gestational diabetes. Maternal factors associated with macrosomia are hyperglycemia, mother being overweight, being obese during pregnancy (>18 kg), advanced maternal age, and multiparity.[35,36] While the rate of women delivering baby over 4,500 g is 2% in the general obstetric population, it is 4% among women with GD diagnosis.[37] It is reported that 20–30% of the infants of women with GD diagnosis but not undergoing treatment born above 4,000 g.[38]

Fetal growth rate increases particularly in the second half of pregnancy. Maternal hyperglycemia (postprandial hyperglycemia in particular) in this period causes fetal hyperinsulinemia and fetal growth is triggered. Macrosomic fetuses of diabetic pregnant women are different anthropometrically from the macrosomic fetuses of normal pregnant women. There is excessive fat accumulation in the shoulders and bodies of these fetuses. This increases the prevalence of shoulder dystocia, brachial plexus injuries, and clavicle fracture.[39] Similarly, cephalopelvic disproportion resulted in cesarean section is more frequent. Macrosomia is closely associated with neonatal hypoglycemia in particular and other metabolic complications in diabetic pregnant women. Unexplained sudden intrauterine death near term and asymmetric septal hypertrophy causing cardiac ventricle dysfunction are more frequent in these infants.[40]

## Shoulder Dystocia and Birth Trauma

Macrosomia causes increase in the prevalence of shoulder dystocia which may result in brachial plexus injury and clavicle fractures in newborns of patients with GD. The prevalence of shoulder dystocia is 6–10 times higher in the infants of diabetic mothers.[1] Brachial plexus injuries may cause a permanent damage in 5–22% of the babies.[41]

## Interventional and Cesarean Deliveries

The rates of interventional and cesarean deliveries have increased depending on macrosomia, intrauterine growth retardation (IUGR) and presentation anomalies. The rate of cesarean is even higher in macrosomic fetuses in cases where glucose control cannot be established adequately. As the diabetes control gets worse, the cesarean rate increases accordingly. The most significant factors here except fetal weight are the failure of labor induction and fetal asphyxia. Cesarean section is recommended in diabetic pregnancies with fetal weights estimated 4,500 g and above.[1] Normal vaginal delivery is recommended in other cases, and applying cervical prostaglandin in cases where labor induction is required is the only logical method to choose.

Timing of delivery is also a problematic issue for diabetic pregnancies. In cases with pregestational diabetes where glucose is well controlled, planning delivery after 39 weeks is suitable.[42] However, either with or without insulin, no safe delivery week has been determined to recommend in the perspective of evidence-based medicine for GD cases.[1] Therefore, 39 weeks of gestation should be aimed as in cases with overt diabetes.

The frequency of fetal well-being tests is quite controversial. In GD cases with well-controlled metabolism, each physician and clinic may decide according to their own practices. However, GD and pregestational diabetes cases with weak glycemic control are under risk in terms of fetal asphyxia and the tests showing fetal well-being should certainly be performed in this group. Tests showing fetal well-being can be begun between 28 weeks and 32 weeks according to the glycemic control medical complications (nephropathy, vasculopathy, etc.) of patients.

## Hypertension—Preeclampsia

They develop particularly during the late periods of pregnancy. While the association between GD and preeclampsia is revealed, the responsible mechanisms are still unclear. It is considered that the endothelial dysfunction in such cases cannot produce prostacyclin (PGI2) sufficient enough to meet elevated angiotensin-2 and vasopressin. It is seen in 5–10% in all pregnancies. Preeclampsia is seen more frequently in diabetic pregnant women with vascular problems such as proteinuria in particular. The increase of perinatal mortality is 20 times higher than those with normal blood pressure and it is considered as the main reason for maternal and fetal loss. While the relationship of insulin resistance with high blood pressure and obesity was shown and this relationship was clearly defined in men and nonpregnant women, the relationship of glucose intolerance with the problems concurrent with hypertension in pregnant women could not be determined with so accurate borders.[43] In the studies performed, mean artery blood pressures of patients whose GD is found in the early periods of pregnancy and requiring insulin treatment were higher than the patients with normal glucose tolerance and are regulated with diet. Also, there are authors claiming that pregnancy-induced hypertension is the clinical reflection of insulin resistance. The relationship between increasing glucose level and the severity of preeclampsia has been shown in the studies performed.[44] This problem is also the main reason of the premature labor in diabetic pregnant women. Today, findings have been accumulating and it is considered that the insulin resistance has a role in the development of preeclampsia, at least partially. It can be also thought that treating insulin resistance with this mechanism will decrease preeclampsia risk and even other anti-inflammatory effects of balancing carbohydrate metabolism of insulin may be protective against the development of preeclampsia. In a meta-analysis including 11 randomized controlled studies, the effects of insulin and metformin treatment were compared and a significant decrease was found in the pregnancy-induced hypertension with metformin treatment. Also, no difference was found in terms of preeclampsia between the groups undergoing insulin or metformin treatment. Therefore, the activities of insulin and metformin were found similar on the prevalence of preeclampsia in terms of treatment activity.[45]

## Polyhydramnios

Polyhydramnios is seen in about one-third of the diabetic pregnancies. In such case, pregnant women should definitely be evaluated in terms of fetal malformations (particularly for the malformations of central nervous system and gastrointestinal system). However, it is considered that the presence of polyhydramnios in diabetic cases does not cause an additional increase in perinatal morbidity or mortality.[46]

## Neonatal Metabolic Disorders

The prevalence of hypoglycemia, hypocalcemia, hypomagnesemia, polycythemia, and hyperbilirubinemia of babies born from women with gestational diabetes.

## Hypoglycemia

The incidence rate of hypoglycemia was found as 25–40%.[47] The incidence rate of hypoglycemia was reported high also in mothers with well-controlled plasma glucose concentration.[48] It is considered that intrapartum glycemic control in particular determines the hypoglycemia risk of newborn. If hypoglycemia is not detected and intervened on time, it may lead to seizure, coma, and brain damage. Therefore, glucose follow-ups should be monitored carefully following the delivery until good metabolic control of the neonate is accomplished.

## Polycythemia and Hyperviscosity

It is seen in 5–10% of diabetic pregnant women. It is closely related with glycemic control. Due to the decrease in oxygenation, erythropoietin levels of the umbilical cords of infants of diabetic mothers are typically high and therefore the rate of polycythemia is increased in such infants.[24] Polycythemia leads to increase in the prevalence of postnatal hyperbilirubinemia and this also causes the increase in phototherapy need.[41] Another potential problem is the tissue damage and ischemia associated with hyperviscosity.[6]

## Neonatal Hypocalcemia and Hyperbilirubinemia

Neonatal hypocalcemia is a problem seen almost in 50% of the infants of diabetic mothers. It usually appears in the first 3 days of life. The incidence of hyperbilirubinemia is two times higher than health pregnancies and found in 25% of the infants of diabetic mothers.[6] Another reason is the preterm labor associated with diabetes.

## POSTNATAL LONG-TERM RISKS

### Long-term Risks in Terms of Mother

Diabetes develops in about half of the women with GD within 22–28 years in the future.[1] How short will the diabetes develop depends on the personal risk factors. Risks such as ethnic group, obesity, age, and polycystic ovarian syndrome cause diabetes to develop faster. The possibility of developing type 2 DM in patients requiring insulin during pregnancy is higher.[49] For example, diabetes develops within 5 years following the pregnancy in 60% of Latin American women.[1]

It was found in the studies performed that those with GD were under risk also in terms of metabolic syndrome, atherosclerosis, and cardiovascular dysfunction after postpartum third month.[50]

Hyperinsulinemia during pregnancy displays 30–50% decrease just after delivery. The decrease slowly continues within following 6–12 weeks. Blood glucose levels return to normal levels in the early postnatal period in most of the patients with GD. Therefore, evaluating patients between postpartum 6 weeks and 12 weeks in terms of glucose metabolism is very important for determining the risk for the development of type 2 DM within following 5–10 years and establishing patient follow-up strategy.[51,52]

## Long-term Risks in Terms of Fetus

The investigators monitoring the infants of diabetic mothers for future diabetes development reported that diabetes develop in such infants 20 times more than the infants of nondiabetic mothers.[42] Obesity prevalence also increased in these infants. The mechanisms of maternal diabetes leading to future obesity in fetus are not known clearly. In a prospective study comparing the infants of GD, type 1 DM, and nondiabetic pregnant women, it was found that more than one-third of the babies born from women with GD were overweight or obese when they reach at the age of 11 years. This rate was found to be two times higher than those delivered by type 1 DM or nondiabetic women.[53,54] Also, as another important point of this study, it was found that the maternal obesity during early pregnancy period is the most significant factor determining the risk for infants of women with GD being overweight at 2, 8, and 11 years old (and therefore the insulin resistance at early period). It was reported that smoking during pregnancy is also associated with the risk for childhood obesity. This result was found independent from GD treatment and macrosomic birth.[54] The results of this study are remarkable for revealing how the preventable reasons of obesity becoming a serious public health issue is important.

In the HAPO study, which is one of the most significant studies on GD performed, the effect of being obese on fetal birth weight was found to be an additional 174 g, it was 339 g in pregnant women who were GD.[55]

Four groups were created in a cohort study investigating the risk factors for metabolic syndrome (obesity, hypertension, dyslipidemia, and glucose intolerance) during childhood.[27] The groups were macrosomic baby and normal glucose tolerance [LGA (large for gestational age) + control)], macrosomic baby and GD (LGA + GD), normal birth weight and normal glucose tolerance (AGA + control), and normal birth weight and GD [AGA (average for gestational age) + GD]. The development of insulin resistance during childhood was found 10 times higher in LGA + GD group. The risk of developing metabolic syndrome at any period was not found to be different in LGA and AGA control group, but it was found 3.6 times higher in LGA + GD group than AGA + GD group.

It was found in the studies performed that the children of women with pregestational and GD had higher rates of attention-deficit hyperactivity disorder and weaker motor functions during school ages. No change was observed in cognitive functions.[6]

## Benefits of Glucose Tests

The purpose of screening tests during pregnancy is not to diagnose but to determine the group under risk. It is still controversial if it is necessary to carry out diabetes screening during pregnancy or not, if it should be done to all pregnant women or only those under risk, and which method will be used for these tests. However, current data with the evidence-based medicine perspective show us that performing screening and diagnostic tests for GD is very significant in order to identify GD and do appropriate management plans, to decrease early period neonatal and maternal morbidities such as macrosomia, shoulder dystocia and preeclampsia, and to determine metabolic syndrome and related risks on time which are expected for mother and infant in the long-term.

Screening and diagnostic tests performed in the second trimester are done according to preferred test or by drinking 75 g liquid containing glucose as a single step test or 50 g and then 100 g if necessary as a two-step test and then evaluating venous plasma blood sample. These tests have no serious maternal or fetal effects. Only certain patients may have problem for consuming hyperosmolar liquid (more distinct in 100 g glucose).[5] Therefore, 75 g glucose tolerance test (GTT) is considered as diagnostic test at a single step.

When test results indicate GD, first the diet-exercise is planned according to the week of gestation and then medical treatment later if necessary. Also, the family should be informed about perinatal risks that are associated with GD and fetal monitorization is required in case of necessity and the increase of prenatal examination frequency.[5] In a study in which the cases with and without screening were modeled, it was shown that performing the test in populations with high GD and type 2 DM prevalence was beneficial for both preventing type 2 DM and costs.[44] Without any significant decrease in the number of patients which are required to be evaluated with laboratory screening method, not screening patients with low risk may lead to overlook some patients with GD.

## Glucose Tests

Maternal venous plasma changes under normal conditions are as follows when performing GTT: preprandial blood glucose (PBG) is between 80 mg/dL and 90 mg/dL. Within approximately 4–5 minutes, the solution containing 75 g glucose is drunk and BG level increases up to 130–140 mg/dL within 30–40 minutes, it decreases slightly below PBG level within 120–150 minutes; at the end of 180 minutes, PBG level is reached.[56,57] In the individuals with normal carbohydrate metabolism, normal glucose levels are reached within about 2 hours. These tests have no risk for fetuses.[5]

It is still debated which screening should be done for GD (screening everyone or risk-based approach) and which test should be used.[58] The reason for this dispute is that there is no distinct definition in the world in terms of the criteria for screening everyone and it is not clear which glucose intolerance case will provide treatment benefit. At this point, screening test should be selected by considering the purposes of screening and cost-benefit balance.

There are publications stating that GD diagnosis is delayed and there are high false results which are about 10–20% by applying 100 g OGGT to those who had abnormal results from 50 g glucose test.[59] There is difference of opinion on the threshold value of 50 g GTT. When threshold value is considered as 140 mg/dL, 3-hour oral glucose tolerance test (OGTT) is performed in 10–15% of cases and GD is detected in 20–40% of the cases who undergo diagnostic test. With 140 mg/dL threshold value, the sensitivity was calculated as 80% and specificity as 90%, and the diagnosis of approximately 20% of the cases are overlooked.[59] In 10% of the cases, serum

**Table 1.1:** Sensitivity and specificity of the methods used in gestational diabetes diagnosis.[60]

| Screening method | Sensitivity (%) | Specificlty (%) |
|---|---|---|
| Risk factors | 50 | 66 |
| Random glucose measurement | 40 | 90 |
| HbA1c | 40 | 90 |
| 50 g GTT (1-hour 140 mg/dL | 59 | 91 |
| 75 g OGTT | 79 | 83 |

(GTT: Glucose tolerance test; OGTT: Oral glucose tolerance test).

glucose level in GTT is between 130 mg/dL and 140 mg/dL. Therefore, when the threshold value is decreased to 130 mg/dL in GTT, the sensitivity of the test increases to 90; however, the number of patients referred to diagnostic tests increases for 60%. In a study conducted in 2002, the sensitivity and specificity values were identified for GD screening methods and these values were given in Table 1.1.[60] Finally, ADA and ACOG (American College of Obstetricians and Gynecologists) recommend glucose threshold value in serum as 140 mg/dL.[1,2]

## Two-Step Glucose Test

Threshold values checked in venous serum and evaluation of 50 g GTT are as below.[1] No diagnostic test is required for 50 g GTT below 140 mg/dL. In this case, negative predictive value is about 85–90%. So, the risk for overlooking GD in glucose values below 140 mg/dL is 10–15%.[1]

If 50 g GTT is between 140 mg/dL and 180 mg/dL, diagnostic 3-hour 100 g OGTT is applied. GD diagnosis is established in case that two of the values are positive in 100 g OGTT: If PBG is above 95 mg/dL, 1-hour BG is above 180 mg/dL, 2-hour BG is above 155 mg/dL, 3-hour BG is above 140 mg/dL, and 50 g GTT is above 180 mg/dL, the patient is directly established GD diagnosis and the treatment is initiated.

## Single-Step Glucose Test

In 2010, IADPSG (International Association of Diabetes and Pregnancy Study Group) recommended new criteria for GD diagnosis. These diagnoses criteria were determined with HAPO study where the results of multinational 25,000 pregnant women were investigated.[61] New IADPSG criteria were mainly prepared by focusing on the perinatal risk of parameters which are above 90 percentile. Accordingly, it is recommended to check PBG and hemoglobin A1c (HbA1c) or spot blood glucose (sBG). If PBG is above 126 mg/dL and HbA1c is above 6.5% or sBG is above 200 mg/dL, it is recommended to consider it as overt diabetes and treat accordingly. If the results are not consistent with overt diabetes, but PBG is above 92 mg/dL yet below 126 mg/dL, it is recommended to treat by considering it as GD. If PBG is below 92 mg/dL, it is recommended to test with 75 g OGTT between 24 weeks and 28 weeks of gestation. The diagnosis criteria of 75 g OGTT can be listed as follows: If at least one of the values below is positive, it is consistent with GD diagnosis: PBG above 92 mg/dL, 1-hour BG above 180 mg/dL, and 2-hour BG above 153 mg/dL.

## Which Glucose Test should We Do?

The IADPSG criteria differ with the recommendation that performing screening in the first trimester according to the algorithms used previously and screening with 75 g OGTT again in the second trimester if the result is negative in the first one.[2] ACOG recommends carrying out screening in the risk group during the first trimester. When IADPSG criteria were applied, the rate of diagnosed GD cases increased to 18% but they were not adopted by ACOG.[1]

Since there was no optimal approach for the diagnosis of gestational diabetes, National Institutes of Health (NIH) held a consensus meeting with the aim of determining the most appropriate diagnostic approach.[32] The results of related 97 studies (6 randomized controlled studies, 63 prospective cohort studies, and 28 retrospective cohort studies) were investigated and continuous and positive relationship was found between increasing glucose values and macrosomia, and between primary cesarean rates and increasing glucose values at 75 g OGTT. 50 g OGTT has higher negative predictive value as well as suboptimal positive predictive values.

It was reported in a prospective randomized controlled study doing cost analysis by comparing single-step and two-step screening that two-step screening is more convenient for cost analysis.[62] The cost difference being not so much, and applying diet-exercise program to a wider pregnancy group providing positive effects not only on glucose levels but also gestational outcomes should not be overlooked.

Since type 2 diabetes is frequently seen in Turkey, it can be tolerated easily and done at a single step and it is also a diagnostic test, applying 75 g OGTT based on single value positivity to all pregnant women should be addressed as the most appropriate approach.

## To Whom and When to Apply Glucose Test?

In the United States of America, it is logical to screen each pregnant woman since they have at least one of the risk factors that may damage balancing carbohydrate metabolism during pregnancy in 90% of pregnant women.[1] Also, there is no risk factor in about 20% of pregnant women found to have GD.[5] As a result of the systematic review done by the United States Preventive Services Task Force (USPSTF), it was stated that it is required to screen everyone after 24 weeks of gestation, but it does not help to screen everyone during early gestation period and that it is more significant to perform risk-based screening during the first antenatal visit.[61]

If the patient has a risk factor for type 2 DM (obesity, BMI $\geq$30 kg/m$^2$, history of GD or damaged glucose metabolism, polycystic ovarian syndrome, etc.), screening during the first prenatal visit would be a logical approach.

Performing PBG evaluation in the risk group during first antenatal visit and 75 g OGTT during 24–26 weeks of gestation if PBG is below 92 mg/dL would be more appropriate. If the first screening is negative or no screening is performed in the early period, the screening should be carried out at 24–28 weeks of gestation.[5]

There are some matters to consider when conducting GTTs (Table 1.2). It is significant to provide an environment close to basic physiological conditions in order to standardize tests and measurements and to rule out other factors.

**Table 1.2:** Points to consider in oral glucose tolerance test.

- The test should be carried out in the morning
- Fasting is required for at least 8 hours and maximum 14 hours
- Patient should be on diet for at least 3 days uninterruptedly (minimum 150 mg carbohydrate daily). If pregnant woman is on a diet poor for carbohydrate before the text, insulin response to the test is less than the expected and false positivity rate increases
- During the text, pregnant woman should be in sitting position and should not make any effort
- Pregnant woman should not smoke for 12 hours before the test
- Patient should rest for 30 minutes before preprandial glucose measurement
- After preprandial glucose measurement, patient should drink 75 g glucose solution within 5 minutes

## What to Do in Pregnant Women Who Cannot Tolerate Oral Glucose Test?

Performing serial glucose measurement would be logical approach in order to rule out hyperglycemic conditions in pregnant women who cannot tolerate standard OGTT.[5] In pregnant women who have risk factors for GD in particular and cannot tolerate screening tests, it is necessary to perform random PBG and postprandial BG measurements. This approach is also convenient for patients who underwent gastric bypass operation.[5] According to the review of Coustan et al. GD risk is very low in pregnant women whose PBG is lower than 85 mg/dL at 24 weeks of gestation.[61] However, additional tests and measurements are required in values above this value.[5]

HbA1c is significant for evaluating treatment activity rather than screening and it gives information about metabolic process for at least 60 days.

## HbA1c

In the studies, a proper threshold value with good sensitivity and specificity during GD screening could not be found for HbA1c. In four different studies conducted on this matter, HbA1c threshold values were found 5.0, 5.3, 5.5, and 7.5, but no clear result was obtained for detecting GD according to these values.[63-66] In the study of Agarwal et al. performed on 442 patients, it was concluded that HbA1c is a weak test for GD screening.[63] The population size in the study of Uncu et al. was 42 pregnant women and it was stated that HbA1c did not provide any additional contribution.[64] Consequently, HbA1C is not recommended as a screening test due to inconsistencies in the standardization, technical problems, lack of wide- availability and high-cost. However, it is accepted as the "golden standard" for the follow-up of glycemic control.

In regions where healthcare service cannot be provided sufficiently, checking PBG between 24 weeks and 28 weeks of gestation can be a practical approach. In a study conducted in China by compiling the data of 15 hospitals where 24,584 pregnant women were screened, it was reported that performing diagnostic 75 g OGTT on pregnant women whose PBG is between 79–90 mg/dL will reduce the requirement of 2-hour diagnostic test by half.[65] However, when applying screening tests, a specific approach should be determined by considering the characteristics of population. It cannot be generalized in this study since ethnical characteristics affect type 2 DM prevalence and also different threshold values were used in the study conducted in China.[67]

## May Glucose Tests be Harmful for Mother and Fetus?

In the studies performed, it was shown that consuming concentrated hyperosmolar glucose solutions for GD screening and diagnostic tests may cause gastrointestinal osmotic imbalance which results with gastric irritation, delay in gastric discharge, nausea, and vomiting in less number of patients.

In a study performed by Agarwal et al., it was reported that 9.8% of 5,142 pregnant women could not complete 100 g OGTT. The major reason for being unable to complete the test was the vomiting of pregnant women. In 2% of the cases, various reasons were found such as children of pregnant women drinking the solution, eating food during test, not giving blood at required times, and being unable to complete test in term of time.[68] It was reported that OGTT has no side effects other than those stated earlier.[5,69]

## 2014 Cochrane Review: Different Results?

In the Cochrane[70] review in 2014 few high quality evidences on the improvement of maternal and neonatal health by GD screening were found based on the data of 3,972 women and 4 studies (Bergus and Murphy, 1992; Murphy et al., 1994; Griffin et al., 2000; Martinez Collado et al., 2003) which were consistent with the criteria among 31 studies.[71-74] These studies were carried out in limited regions. When thinking on GD risk and screening approach, the characteristics of the population investigated (such as ethnic group, nourishment habits, etc.) should be considered and interpreted accordingly. It would be useful to assess carefully these studies included in 2014 Cochrane review by considering their weak aspects and to remain distant towards the results and interpretations of this review in the current situation.

Since these four studies included in this meta-analysis have included only a particular group of pregnant population with GD, we would recommend further subgroup analysis with sufficient power in order to achieve a more definitive conclusion. Also, other studies are required for determining the efficacy of other methods (such as capillary blood sugar test, glycosuria, etc.) which can be used instead of GTTs that are applied simpler yet cannot be tolerated by some patients.[70]

## HAPO Study: Why Important?

The Hyperglycemia and Adverse Pregnancy Outcome (HAPO) Study is an epidemiological research designed to seek an answer about how various levels of glucose intolerance affects fetal and perinatal outcomes during pregnancies. It is a study planned internationally and including 25,505 pregnant women from various ethnical groups. Its primary results were determined as macrosomia, primary cesarean frequency, neonatal hypoglycemia, and hyperinsulinemia. Preterm labor, preeclampsia, newborn intense care need, shoulder dystocia, birth trauma, and neonatal adiposity were considered as secondary results.[75] A continuous relationship was found between glucose levels below maternal diabetes limits and perinatal outcomes such as birth weight and umbilical cord C-peptide levels. While there is no particular threshold glucose level in predicting gestational outcomes, it was found that there is a direct association with gestational outcomes and complications as preprandial or 1-hour and 2-hour glucose levels increase (even within normal limits). Even though the outcomes of this study are below overt diabetes levels, the more blood glucose levels are kept under control, the more it reflects positively to the gestational outcomes.

However, observing poor gestational outcomes also in pre- and postprandial blood glucose levels that we identified within "normal" levels make us consider that new threshold values should be used in screening models. In the light of the results of HAPO study, new IADPSG criteria were defined.[76] While single positive value being sufficient for the diagnosis and also the threshold values being slightly lower increase the sensitivity in the new IADPSG criteria, the prevalence of diagnosed GD cases increases to 18%.[1] These threshold values correspond to mean glucose levels where birth weight, umbilical cord C-peptide levels, and macrosomia risk increase 1.75 times. In cases established with GD diagnosis according to these threshold values, macrosomia, preeclampsia, and preterm labor risks increase 2 times. However, further studies are needed to get more information how gestational outcomes will improve or if they will improve or not depending on the treatment in GD cases diagnosed according to IADPSG criteria. It was observed that perinatal complications decreased from 4% to 1% in the study of Crowther et al. for randomized treatment activity on control group and the cases diagnosed with 75 g OGTT during 24–28 weeks. It was found that glucose control, diet, and treatment program with insulin in required cases decreased perinatal morbidity significantly.[48] A similar randomized study was conducted by Landon et al. on a milder case group in 2009.[77] In that study, 50 g and 100 g glucose tests were used during 24–31 weeks of gestation on pregnant group who had abnormal values in tests but the level of preprandial BG was below 95 g. While perinatal losses (no perinatal death case) and severe newborn complications did not decrease with the treatment program applied in this study, a particular improvement was observed in the rates of birth weight, shoulder dystocia, cesarean, and preeclampsia. Finding treatment activity even in mild cases with this study shows that glucose level and perinatal outcomes are directly associated even without a particular threshold value of HAPO study.[75] While the rates of cases diagnosed with GD increased twice by using 75 g and single value seem as an advantage, they seem as an advantage assessing the results of Landon et al. study.[77]

The direct association between perinatal outcomes and glucose level found in HAPO study (also in low glucose level) shows the significance and efficiency of diet-exercise program. In this sense, applying 75 g and single value OGTT to all pregnant women doubles the rates of GD but it also helps to apply diet-exercise program to pregnant women and therefore to improve perinatal outcomes. Although its activity on short-term outcomes was revealed by the studies published by Crowther et al.[48] and Landon et al.,[77] there has been no study showing its activity on long-term outcomes. It will become clearer with further studies to be performed on the activity of this new diagnosis and treatment approach.

It was shown in a study investigating the effects of high pregestational maternal body mass index on gestational outcomes that pregestational BMI is related with more operative delivery and more neonatal problems.[78] GD prevalence was found as 21.1% in the study of Göymen et al.[79] It was claimed in the same study that there was no difference in terms of GD rates when two-step or single-step screening is performed.[79] In a study investigating maternal serum leptin and malondialdehyde (MDA) levels in GD diagnosis and screening, it was reported that leptin, MDA, and HbA1c levels increased significantly in GD cases, and these tests were found to increase the specificity of the GD screening modalities.[80] In another study comparing maternal serum adiponectin and leptin measurements in GD diagnosis and screening, it was shown that adiponectin was more sensitive but had equal specificity in the group which underwent 75 g OGTT. Adiponectin was found significantly low in the group which underwent two-step screening.[81]

In a study evaluating 50 g screening and 100 g OGTT results of 690 pregnant women in terms of fetal macrosomia, it was argued that the patients with 50 g screening result over 140 mg/dL should be followed up closely in terms of fetal macrosomia like the patients with GD even though their 100 g OGTT results are not positive.[82] In another study investigating the etiological factors in macrosomic fetuses, maternal age being above 35, high parity, high average of maternal height, weight gained during pregnancy being over 12 kg, high level of HbA1c, presence of polyhydramnios in current pregnancy, and the medical history with macrosomic infant were considered as the factors increasing macrosomia risk in fetus.[83]

## TYPE 1/TYPE 2 DIABETES DURING PREGNANCY

Diabetes is the disorder of carbohydrate metabolism affecting life considerably. It is a chronic disease leading long-term complications such as retinopathy, nephropathy, and vascular diseases. It is seen in 2–5% of women in England. While 5% of this group is type 2 DM, type 1 DM is 7.5% and GD is 87.5%. It is known that the rates of type 1 and type 2 diabetes gradually increase. Type 2 diabetes is frequently seen in Africa, Caribbean, South Asia, Middle East, and China in particular.[6-8]

Miscarriage, preeclampsia, and early labor are seen frequently in diabetic pregnant women (type 1 and type 2). Besides, it should be remembered that retinopathy may get worse during pregnancy. Postpartum compliance problems such as stillbirth, congenital anomalies, macrosomia, birth trauma, perinatal mortality, and hypoglycemia are seen more frequently.[22,23,31]

One of the first steps of making a successful follow-up in diabetic patients is to establish a good communication between healthcare professionals and patient. It is useful to provide detailed information on diabetes and pregnancy as well as delivering this information to patient in written. In this way, patient has a referring source when required. Diabetic (type 1 or type 2) pregnant women can be clinically taken care of as in Table 1.3.

## CONCLUSION AND RECOMMENDATIONS

The 75 g OGTT at 24–28 weeks of gestation on routine base in low risk group is recommended for the diagnosis of gestational diabetes. The direct association between perinatal outcomes and glucose level, and also the significance and efficiency of diet-exercise program have been recently shown in many studies. In this sense, applying 75 g and single value OGTT to all pregnant women doubles the rates of GD but it also helps to apply diet-exercise program to

**Table 1.3:** Recommendation for the management of diabetes in pregnancy.

*Before pregnancy:*

- Patient should be informed about the importance of regulating glucose level well before pregnancy and also maintaining this level after pregnancy. In this way, the awareness that it is possible to prevent miscarriage, congenital malformation, stillbirth, and newborn death should be raised
    - Significance of diet, weight, and exercise
    - Hypoglycemia developing during pregnancy
    - How nausea-vomiting during pregnancy may affect glucose control
    - How the condition of large for gestational age may increase birth trauma, labor induction, and cesarean possibilities
    - How it is important to manage the condition of diabetic retinopathy before (treating if necessary) and during pregnancy
    - The importance of maintaining glucose level well during labor in order to prevent newborn hypoglycemia and providing early lactation of infant after birth
    - Conditions which may develop and require special or intense care in infant after birth even temporarily.
- It should be informed in detail to such patients beginning from adolescence period that an unplanned pregnancy would be an undesired condition and it is very significant to conduct a well-planned birth control and if it will be discontinued, to refer to doctor and make a pregestational plan
- Diabetic patients planning pregnancy should be informed that:
    - Risks associated with diabetes during pregnancy is also associated with diabetes period
    - It is important to conduct conception until a well glucose control (HbA1c being below 6.1%) is provided
    - Glucose level targets, glucose monitoring, treatment options if necessary, and treatment options for problems associated with diabetes and pregnancy should be discussed
    - A closer cooperation is required during pregnancy and management plans such as emergency cases should be discussed in details
    - Diet should be arranged for those planning to get pregnant
    - Weight loss program should be applied and informed about its significance for those planning to get pregnant and have BMI above 27 kg/m$^2$
    - It is important to have 5 mg/day folic acid certainly by those planning to get pregnant in order to decrease the risk for neural tube defect
    - It is very important to do glucose measurements by themselves and they should be recorded by times
    - Type 1 diabetics in particular have to do ketonuria check with sticks when their glucose levels elevate or when they do not feel well

*Reliability of diabetic drugs during pregnancy:*

- They should be informed that metformin used alone or as a support for insulin is an effective drug to get glucose levels. Other diabetic drugs should be discontinued before pregnancy and insulin should be used instead
- It should be known that it was not shown in clinical studies that rapid-acting insulin analogs (aspart or lispro) used during pregnancy have negative effects on fetus or newborn

*Contd...*

*Contd…*

- It should be stated to those undergoing insulin treatment or planning to get pregnant that there is insufficient data on the use of long-acting insulin analogs during pregnancy and therefore NPH (neutral protamine Hagedorn) insulin has been still an option preferred

Treatment reliability of diabetic complications during pregnancy:

- Angiotensin-converting enzyme inhibitors and angiotensin-2 receptor antagonists should be discontinued before pregnancy or they should be discontinued as soon as possible when pregnancy is detected. Instead, other alternative treatments should be performed
- Statins should be discontinued as soon as possible when pregnancy is detected

Retina evaluation before pregnancy:

- Diabetic patients are absolutely required to have retina examination before pregnancy (if it is not performed within last 6 months)
- It is useful to perform this examination first by drop and then digital imaging

Renal examination before pregnancy:

- It is significant to examine kidneys including microalbuminuria before discontinuing birth control. If creatinine is ≥120 or glomerular filtration rate is <45, it should be reevaluated after nephrology consultation

*Glucose follow-up in gestation*:

- Where possible, preprandial glucose level should be kept about 65–95 mg/dL and 1-hour glucose below 140 mg/dL, and importance of these levels should be explained
- Patients with overt diabetes using insulin should be informed about the possibility of hypoglycemia attacks during first trimester in particular and the precautions
- The cases whose glucose levels cannot be managed despite insulin use should be explained that using insulin pump is another method
- Conditions where diabetic ketoacidosis is in question should be evaluated in hospital immediately and they should be put under care
- It should be explained that diabetic retinopathy does not inhibit vaginal labor
- It should be explained to pregnant women with overt diabetes that they should visit for diabetes control with 1–2 weeks of interval

*Gestational follow-up*:

- First examination: Explaining the importance of and teaching glucose control, detailed anamnesis check for diabetes, drugs used, retina/kidney assessment
- Evaluating pregnancy at 7–9 weeks of gestation
- 13–14 weeks of fetal anatomy and fetal ECHO examination, diabetes and gestational interactions, delivery and lactation and newborn information
- Reevaluating if retinopathy or nephropathy is found
- Fetal anatomy and fetal ECHO examination at 20–22 weeks of gestation
- Fetal development and amniotic fluid examination at 28 weeks of gestation, recheck if retinopathy or nephropathy is not detected in the first examination
- Fetal development and amniotic fluid check at 32 weeks of gestation
- Informing about fetal growth and amniotic fluid examination at 36 weeks of gestation, delivery timing-method and delivery management, analgesia or anesthesia, labor and then hypoglycemia management, infant care after delivery, lactation and its effect on glucose control, and conception

*Contd…*

*Contd...*

- Unless there is fetal growth retardation, it is not necessary to do fetal well-being test routinely in diabetic pregnant women before 38 weeks of gestation
- Fetal well-being tests in pregnant woman with approaching delivery at 38 weeks and inducting labor or planning cesarean if necessary
- Fetal well-being tests at 39 weeks of in gestational diabetes
- Fetal well-being tests at 40 weeks of gestational diabetes
- Fetal well-being tests at 41 weeks of gestational diabetes

*Preterm labor:*
- Checking if diabetes constitutes contraindication for the administration of steroid or tocolysis (without using beta mimetics) if necessary
- Additional insulin will be required if steroid is administered, and glucose check should be performed more strictly

*Timing and management of delivery:*
- In cases with normal fetal growth, delivery can be done by labor induction after 38 weeks of gestation and if necessary, cesarean can be planned
- If fetal macrosomia is in question, pregnant woman should be informed about the risks of vaginal delivery, labor induction, and cesarean
- In diabetic pregnant women, it would be beneficial to carry out evaluation and inform in terms of anesthesia in third trimester
- If general anesthesia is applied, it should be known that glucose check is required every 30 minutes and it should be monitored until the effect of anesthesia diminish after delivery

*Managing labor:*
- Capillary glucose level should be checked every hour during labor and it should be kept at 75–125 mg/dL
- Applying dextrose infusion as well as insulin as of the onset of labor
- If glucose level cannot be maintained at 75–125 mg/dL also in other cases, applying insulin together with dextrose infusion

*Newborn management:*
- Diabetic pregnant women should deliver in a hospital capable of newborn resuscitation for 24 hours
- Babies of diabetic mothers should be kept near their mothers. If any clinical complication or abnormal finding develops, then they should be monitored under special or intense care conditions
- Glucose control of the infants of diabetic mothers should be performed every 2–4 hours routinely and if there is any clinical finding, they should be controlled for polycythemia, hyperbilirubinemia, hypocalcemia and hypomagnesemia
- If there is any cardiomyopathy finding including congenital cardiac anomaly or murmur, fetal ECHO should be carried out
- Infants of diabetic mothers with following findings should be monitored in newborn intense care units:
  - Hypoglycemia with clinical finding
  - Respiratory distress
  - Cardiomyopathy or cardiac failure due to congenital cardiac anomaly
  - Newborn encephalopathy

*Contd...*

*Contd…*

- – Polycythemia finding (need for partial blood exchange)
- – Intravenous fluid need
- – Need for gavage
- – Need for intense phototherapy and bilirubin control
- – Those born before 34 weeks.
- Each obstetrics clinic should have and provide written information form for preventing, identifying, and managing newborn hypoglycemia
- Despite all kinds of efforts, if blood glucose level decreases below 36 mg in two consecutive measurements and if there is any abnormal clinical finding, gavage or intravenous dextrose application should be performed
- If clinical finding of hypoglycemia is observed, glucose control should be performed immediately and dextrose should be rapidly administered intravenously
- Newborns of diabetic mothers should be fed right after delivery (within 30 minutes) and then every 2–3 hours
- Those with type 2 diabetes may continue using metformin but other drugs should not be used during lactation
- The drugs for diabetic complications discontinued before and during pregnancy should be continued

*Effects of lactation on glucose control*:

- Those with overt diabetes should decrease insulin doses right after delivery and they should be managed with frequent glucose control until the optimum level is obtained
- Those with overt diabetes and using insulin should be informed that hypoglycemia risk will increase after delivery and they should keep available food or snack as they may be required before and after lactation
- If those with gestational diabetes are using drug, they should discontinue their treatment right after delivery

*Postpartum follow-up and information*:

- After delivery, those with overt diabetes should be referred to the clinic that they are followed up
- The glucose levels with gestational diabetes after delivery should be checked before discharging
- Those with gestational diabetes should be warned and informed about the risk for developing hypoglycemia
- Those with gestational diabetes should be checked for weight during postpartum period, diet-exercise applications should be maintained and their preprandial glucose levels should be checked at 6 weeks (not OGTT)
- Those with gestational diabetes should be warned and informed that they may be diabetic later. They should undergo preprandial blood glucose check or OGTT in advance when they plan pregnancy.

(OGTT: Oral glucose tolerance test)

pregnant women and therefore to improve perinatal outcomes. Although its activity on short-term outcomes was revealed by the studies. There has been no study showing its activity on long-term outcomes. It will become clearer with further studies to be performed on the activity of this new diagnosis and treatment approach.

# REFERENCES

1. Committee on Practice Bulletins—Obstetrics. Practice Bulletin No. 137: Gestational diabetes mellitus. Obstet Gynecol. 2013;122:406-16.
2. International Association of Diabetes and Pregnancy Study Groups Consensus Panel; Metzger BE, Gabbe SG, Persson B, Buchanan TA, et al. International association of diabetes and pregnancy study groups recommendations on the diagnosis and classification of hyperglycemia in pregnancy. Diabetes Care. 2010;33(3):676-82.
3. World Health Organization. Diagnostic criteria and classification of hyperglycaemia first detected in pregnancy. Geneva: World Health Organization; 2013.
4. American Diabetes Association. Diagnosis and classification of diabetes mellitus. Diabetes Care. 2014;37 Suppl 1:S81-90.
5. Coustan DR, Jovanovic L. Diabetes mellitus in pregnancy: screening and diagnosis. In: Nathan DM, Greene MN, Barrs VA (Eds). 2014. [online] UpToDate website. Available from: www.uptodate.com [Accessed July 2017].
6. Moore TR, Hauguel-De Mouzon S, Catalano P. Diabetes in pregnancy. In: Creasy RK, Resnik R, Greene MF, et al (Eds). Creasy and Resnik's Maternal-fetal Medicine: Principles and Practice, 7th edition. Philadelphia, PA: Saunders-Elsevier; 2014. pp. 988-1021.
7. Ferrara A. Increasing prevalence of gestational diabetes mellitus: a public health perspective. Diabetes Care. 2007;30 Suppl 2:S141-S6.
8. Centers for Disease Control and Prevention. National Diabetes Statistics Report: estimates of diabetes and its burden in the United States, 2014. Atlanta, GA: U.S. Department of Health and Human Services; 2014.
9. Petraglia F, D'Antona D. Maternal endocrine and metabolic adaptation to pregnancy. In: Lockwood CJ, Snyder PJ, Eckler K (Eds). 2014. [online] UpToDate website. Available from: www.uptodate.com [Accessed July 2017].
10. Solomon CG, Willett WC, Carey VJ, et al. A prospective study of pregravid determinants of gestational diabetes mellitus. JAMA. 1997;278:1078-83.
11. Chasan-Taber L. Gestational diabetes: is it preventable? Am J Lifestyle Med. 2012;6:395-406.
12. Hedderson MM, Darbinian JA, Quesenberry CP, et al. Pregravid cardiometabolic risk profile and risk for gestational diabetes mellitus. Am J Obstet Gynecol. 2011;205:55.e1-7.
13. Moller DE. Potential role of TNF-alpha in the pathogenesis of insulin resistance and type 2 diabetes. Trends Endocrinol Metab. 2000;11:212-7.
14. Bao W, Min D, Twigg SM, et al. Monocyte CD147 is induced by advanced glycation end products and high glucose concentration: possible role in diabetic complications. Am J Physiol Cell Physiol. 2010;299:1212-9.
15. Artunc-Ulkumen B, Pala HG, Pala EE, et al. Exenatide improves ovarian and endometrial injury and preserves ovarian reserve in streptozocin induced diabetic rats. Gynecol Endocrinol. 2015;31:196-201.
16. Dandona P, Aljada A, Bandyopadhyay A. Inflammation: the link between insulin resistance, obesity and diabetes. Trends Immunol. 2004;25:4-7.
17. Satman I, Omer B, Tutuncu Y, et al.; TURDEP-II Study Group. Twelve years trends in the prevalence and risk factors of diabetes and prediabetes in Turkish adults. Eur J Epidemiol. 2013;28:169-80.
18. Satman I, Yilmaz T, Sengül A, et al. Population-based study of diabetes and risk characteristics in Turkey: results of the Turkish diabetes epidemiology study (TURDEP). Diabetes Care. 2002;25:1551-6.
19. International Diabetes Federation (IDF). Diabetes Atlas, 6th edition. Brussels, Belgium: International Diabetes Federation; 2013.
20. Danilenko-Dixon DR, Van Winter JT, Nelson RL, et al. Universal versus selective gestational diabetes screening: application of 1997 American Diabetes Association recommendations. Am J Obstet Gynecol. 1999;181:798-812.

21. Horvath K, Koch K, Jeitler K, et al. Effects of treatment in women with gestational diabetes mellitus: systematic review and meta-analysis. BMJ. 2010;340:c1395.
22. Jovanovic L, Knopp RH, Kim H, et al. Elevated pregnancy losses at high and low extremes of maternal glucose in early normal and diabetic pregnancy: evidence for a protective adaptation in diabetes. Diabetes Care. 2005;28:1113-7.
23. Schwartz R, Grupposo PA, Petzold K, et al. Hyperinsulinemia and macrosomia in the fetus of the diabetic mother. Diabetes Care. 1994;17:640-8.
24. Widness JA, Teramo KA, Clemons GK, et al. Direct relationship of antepartum glucose control and fetal erythropoietin in human type 1 (insulin-dependent) diabetic pregnancy. Diabetologia. 1990;33:378-83.
25. Cordero L, Treuer SH, Landon MB, et al. Management of infants of diabetic mothers. Arch Pediatr Adolesc Med. 1998;152:249-54.
26. Pettitt DJ, Lawrence JM, Beyer J, et al. Association between maternal diabetes in utero and age at offspring's diagnosis of type 2 diabetes. Diabetes Care. 2008;32:2126-30.
27. Boney CM, Verma A, Tucker R, et al. Metabolic syndrome in childhood: association with birth weight, maternal obesity and gestational diabetes mellitus. Pediatrics. 2005;115:e290-6.
28. Pettitt DJ, Knowler WC, Baird HR, et al. Gestational diabetes: infant and maternal complications of pregnancy in relation to third-trimester glucose tolerance in the Pima Indians. Diabetes Care. 1980;3:458.29.
29. Evers IM, de Valk HW, Visser GH. Risk of complications of pregnancy in women with type 1 diabetes: nationwide prospective study in the Netherlands. BMJ. 2004;328:915.
30. Landon MB, Mele L, Spong CY, et al. Eunice Kennedy Shriver National Institute of Child Health, and Human Development (NICHD) Maternal–Fetal Medicine Units (MFMU) Network. The relationship between maternal glycemia and perinatal outcome. Obstet Gynecol. 2011;117:218-24.
31. Sibai BM, Caritis S, Hauth J, et al. Risks of preeclampsia and adverse neonatal outcomes among women with pregestational diabetes mellitus. National Institute of Child Health and Human Development Network of Maternal-Fetal Medicine Units. Am J Obstet Gynecol. 2000;182:364-9.
32. National Institutes of Health consensus development conference statement: diagnosing gestational diabetes mellitus, March 4-6, 2013. Obstet Gynecol. 2013;122:358-69.
33. Centers for Disease Control (CDC). Perinatal mortality and congenital malformations in infants born to women with insulin-dependent diabetes mellitus-United States, Canada, and Europe, 1940-1988. MMWR Morb Mortal Wkly Rep. 1990;39:363-5.
34. Whitelaw B, Gayle C. Gestational diabetes. Obstet Gynaecol Reprod Med. 2011;21:41-6.
35. Caughey AB. Gestational diabetes mellitus: obstetrical issues and management. In: Greene MF, Barss VA (Eds). 2014. [online] UpToDate website. Available from: www.uptodate.com [Accessed July 2017].
36. Hillier TA, Pedula KL, Vesco KK, et al. Excess gestational weight gain: modifying fetal macrosomia risk associated with maternal glucose. Obstet Gynecol. 2008;112:1007-14.
37. Ales KL, Santini DL. Should all pregnant women be screened for gestational glucose intolerance? Lancet. 1989;1(8648):1187-91.
38. Garner P, Okun N, Keely E, et al. A randomized controlled trial of strict glycemic control and tertiary level obstetric care versus routine obstetric care in the management of gestational diabetes: a pilot study. Am J Obstet Gynecol. 1997;177:190-5.
39. McFarland MB, Trylovich CG, Langer O. Anthropometric differences in macrosomic infants in diabetic and nondiabetic mothers. J Matern Fetal Med. 1998;7:292-5.
40. Kenzel W, Misselwitz B. Unexpected fetal death during pregnancy-a problem of unrecognized fetal disorders during antenatal care. Eur J Obstet Gynecol Reprod Biol. 2003;110 Suppl 1:86-92.
41. Hollander MH, Paarlberg KM, Huisjes AJM. Gestational diabetes: a review of the current literature and guidelines. Obstet Gynecol Surv. 2007;62:125-39.
42. Witkop CT, Neale D, Wilson LM, et al. Active compared with expectant delivery management in women with gestational diabetes: a systematic review. Obstet Gynecol. 2009;113:206-17.
43. Berkowitz KM. Insulin resistance and preeclampsia. Clin Perinatol. 1998;25:873-85.

44. Yogev Y, Xenakis EM, Langer O. The association between preeclampsia and the severity of gestational diabetes: the impact of glycemic control. Am J Obstet Gynecol. 2004;191:1655-60.
45. Li G, Zhao S, Cui S, et al. Effect comparison of metformin with insulin treatment for gestational diabetes: a meta-analysis based on RCTs. Arch Gynecol Obstet. 2015;292:111-20.
46. Shoham I, Wiznitzer A, Silberstein T, et al. Gestational diabetes complicated by hydramnios was not associated with increased risk of perinatal morbidity and mortality. Eur J Obstet Gynecol Reprod Biol. 2001;100:46-9.
47. Casey BM, Lucas MJ, MCIntire DD, et al. Pregnancy outcomes in women with gestational diabetes compared with the general obstetric population. Obstet Gynecol. 1997;90:869-73.
48. Crowther CA, Hiller JE, Moss JR, et al. Australian Carbohydrate Intolerance Study in Pregnant Women (ACHOIS) Trial Group. Effect of treatment of gestational diabetes mellitus on pregnancy outcomes. N Engl J Med. 2005;352:2477-83.
49. Tamas G, Kerenyi Z. Current controversies in the mechanisms and treatment of gestational diabetes. Curr Diab Rep. 2002;2:337-46.
50. Coustan DR. Gestational diabetes mellitus: glycemic control and maternal prognosis. In: Nathan DM, Greene MN, Barrs VA (Eds). 2014. [online] UpToDate website. Available from: www.uptodate.com [Accessed July 2017].
51. Gaudier FL, Hauth JC, Poist M, et al. Recurrence of gestational diabetes mellitus. Obstet Gynecol. 1992;80:755-8.
52. American Diabetes Association. 12. Management of diabetes in pregnancy. Diabetes Care. 2016;39 Suppl 1:S94–98.
53. Kim C, Newton KM, Knopp RH. Gestational diabetes and the incidence of type 2 diabetes: a systematic review. Diabetes Care. 2002;25(10):1862-8.
54. Boerschmann H, Pflüger M, Henneberger L, et al. Prevalence and predictors of overweight and insulin resistance in offspring of mothers with gestational diabetes mellitus. Diabetes Care. 2010;33:845-9.
55. McIntyre HD, Cruickshank JK, McCance DR, et al. HAPO Study Cooperative Research Group. The hyperglycemia and adverse pregnancy outcome study: associations of GDM and obesity with pregnancy outcomes. Diabetes Care. 2012;35:780-6.
56. Vasudevan DM, Sreekumari S, Vaidyanathan K. Regulation of blood glucose, insulin and diabetes mellitus. In: Vasudevan DM, Sreekumari S, Vaidyanathan K (Eds). Textbook of Biochemistry for Medical Student. Section C: Clinical and Applied Biochemistry, 7th edition. New Delhi: Jaypee Brothers Publishers; 2013. pp. 311-34.
57. Paulev PE, Zubieta-Calleja. Blood glucose and diabetes. In: Paulev PE, Zubieta-Calleja G (Eds). New Human Physiology. Textbook in Medical Physiology and Pathophysiology: Essentials and Clinical Problems, 2nd edition. Copenhagen: University of Copenhagen; 2004.
58. Coustan D, Nelson C, Carpenter MW, et al. Maternal age and screening for gestational diabetes: a population-based study. Obstet Gynecol. 1989;73:557-61.
59. Ray R, Heng BH, Lim C, et al. Gestational diabetes in Singaporean women: use of the glucose challenge test as a screening test and identification of high risk factors. Ann Acad Med Singapore. 1996;25:504-8.
60. Hana FW, Peters JR. Screening for gestational diabetes; past, present and future. Diabet Med. 2002;19:351-8.
61. Moyer VA; U.S. Preventive Services Task Force. Screening for gestational diabetes mellitus: U.S. Preventive Services Task Force recommendation statement. Ann Intern Med. 2014;160: 414-20.
62. Meltzer SJ, Snyder J, Penrod JR, et al. Gestational diabetes mellitus screening and diagnosis: a prospective randomized controlled trial comparing costs of one-step and two-step methods. BJOG. 2010;117:407-15.
63. Agarwal MM, Hughes PF, Punnose J, et al. Gestational diabetes screening of a multiethnic, high-risk population using glycated proteins. Diabetes Res Clin Pract. 2001;51:67-73.

64. Uncu G, Ozan H, Cengiz C. The comparison of 50 grams glucose challenge test, HbA1c and fructosamine levels in diagnosis of gestational diabetes mellitus. Clin Exp Obstet Gynecol. 1995;22:230-4.
65. Agarwal MM, Dhatt GS, Punnose J, et al. Gestational diabetes: a reappraisal of HBA1c as a screening test. Acta Obstet Gynecol Scand. 2005;84:1159-63.
66. Rajput R, Yogesh Yadav, Rajput M, et al. Utility of HbA1c for diagnosis of gestational diabetes mellitus. Diabetes Res Clin Pract. 2012;98:104-7.
67. Zhu WW, Fan L, Yang HX, et al. Fasting plasma glucose at 24-28 weeks to screen for gestational diabetes mellitus: new evidence from China. Diabetes Care. 2013;36:2038-40.
68. Agarwal MM, Punnose J, Dhatt GS. Gestational diabetes: problems associated with the oral glucose tolerance test. Diabetes Res Clin Pract. 2004;63:73-4.
69. Linder K, Schleger F, Ketterer C, et al. Maternal insulin sensitivity is associated with oral glucose-induced changes in fetal brain activity. Diabetologia. 2014;57:1192-8.
70. Tieu J, McPhee AJ, Crowther CA, et al. Screening and subsequent management for gestational diabetes for improving maternal and infant health. Cochrane Database Syst Rev. 2014;2:CD007222.
71. Bergus GR, Murphy NJ. Screening for gestational diabetes mellitus: comparison of a glucose polymer and a glucose monomer test beverage. J Am Board Fam Pract. 1992;5:241-7.
72. Murphy NJ, Meyer BA, O'Kell RT, et al. Carbohydrate sources for gestational diabetes screening. A comparison. J Reprod Med. 1994;39:977-81.
73. Griffin ME, Coffey M, Johnson H, et al. Universal vs. risk factor-based screening for gestational diabetes mellitus: detection rates, gestation at diagnosis and outcome. Diab Med. 2000;17:26-32.
74. Martinez Collado JH, Alvarado Gay FJ, DaneL Beltran JA, et al. Glucose screening test in pregnant women. A comparison between the traditional glucose load and diet. Medicina Interna de Mexico. 2003;19:286-8.
75. HAPO Study Cooperative Research Group. The Hyperglycemia and Adverse Pregnancy Outcome (HAPO) Study. Int J Gynecol Obstet. 2002;78:69-77.
76. Lowe LP, Metzger BE, Dyer AR, et al.; HAPO Study Cooperative Research Group. Hyperglycemia and Adverse Pregnancy Outcome (HAPO) Study: associations of maternal A1C and glucose with pregnancy outcomes. Diabetes Care. 2012;35:574-80.
77. Landon MB, Spong CY, Thom E, et al. Eunice Kennedy Shriver National Institute of Child Health and Human Development Maternal-Fetal Medicine Units Network. A multicenter, randomized trial of treatment for mild gestational diabetes. N Engl J Med. 2009;361:1339-48.
78. Dündar Ö, Çiftpınar T, Tütüncü L, et al. The effects of the pre-pregnancy maternal body mass index on the pregnancy outcomes. Perinatal Journal. 2008;16:43-8.
79. Göymen A, Altınok T, Uludag S, et al. The role of maternal serum adiponectin levels in screening and diagnosis of gestational diabetes mellitus. Perinatal Journal. 2008;16:49-55.
80. Öncül M, Uludag S, Sen C, et al. The role of maternal serum leptin and malondialdehyde levels in screening and diagnosis of gestational diabetes mellitus. Perinatal Journal. 2009;17:1-35.
81. Göymen A, Öncül M, Güralp O, et al. comparison of maternal serum adiponectin and leptin measurements in screening and diagnosis of gestational diabetes mellitus. Perinatal Journal. 2008;16:92-9.
82. Keskin U, Ercan CM, Güngör S, et al. The effects of gestational diabetes mellitus screening and diagnostic tests on fetal macrosomia. Perinatal Journal. 2013;21:133-7.
83. Akyol A, Talay H, Gedikbası A, et al. The factors effective on the macrosomic deliveries of nondiabetic pregnant women. Perinatal Journal. 2014;22:83-7.

# Chapter 2

# General Aspects of Diabetes in Pregnancy

*Sertac Esin, Cihat Sen*

## INTRODUCTION

Diabetes mellitus (DM) may be defined as inability to produce or use sufficient exogenous insulin and carbohydrate intolerance of variable severity with onset or recognition during the present pregnancy is referred as gestational diabetes mellitus (GDM).[1] All over the world, the prevalence of obesity as well as GDM is increasing. Diabetes in pregnancy may be hazardous due to risks to the fetus and pregnant woman. This chapter provides an overview of pregestational and gestational DM, including the epidemiology and pathophysiology of DM, preconceptional, antenatal, birth and postnatal care issues, neonatal-childhood and adult diabetic complications and as well as public health implications.

## CLASSIFICATION AND PHYSIOLOGY

Diabetes mellitus encompasses a group of metabolic diseases and is characterized by chronic hyperglycemia that results from defects in insulin action, insulin secretion, or both. Insulin is an anabolic hormone and defects in secretion or action leads to metabolic disturbances in carbohydrate, lipid, and protein levels. A low level of insulin usually results from defective pancreatic insulin secretion and resistance at target tissues such as adipose tissue, skeletal muscles, and liver or from defects at insulin receptors, signal transduction systems, functional enzymes, and responsible genes leads to insulin resistance. The severity of symptoms in diabetes depends on the type and duration of the disease.

Type 1 DM constitutes 5–10% of DM subjects.[2] It is mainly caused by autoimmune destruction of the pancreatic β cells through humoral (B cell) response and T-cell mediated inflammatory response which results in absolute insulin deficiency.[3] Type 1 DM may be further classified according to the presence of autoimmune antibodies. In type 1A DM, islet cell antibodies or other islet autoantibodies [autoantibodies to insulin (IAA), glutamic acid decarboxylase (GAD, GAD65), protein tyrosine phosphatase (IA2 and IA2β), and zinc transporter protein (ZnT8A)] are present and indicate immune-mediated pathogenesis.[4,5] Some patients do not have pancreatic antibodies or any cause for β-cell destruction, and yet have absolute insulin deficiency. These patients are classified as idiopathic or type 1B DM. Genetic susceptibility, a diabetogenic trigger and/or exposure to a driving antigen may also have a role in β-cell destruction.

Type 2 DM is characterized by hyperglycemia resulting from insulin resistance and relative insulin deficiency. It is commonly associated with obesity, sedentary lifestyle as well as genetic or environmental influences and accompanied by hypertension, high low-density-lipoprotein cholesterol, and low high-density-lipoprotein cholesterol levels. Type 2 DM represents a complex interaction of genes and environmental factors. Insulin resistance becomes more severe with increasing age and weight. Insulin resistance is the hallmark of type 2 DM and may be associated with adipokines secreted by adipocytes, hyperglycemia itself, impaired insulin processing, and islet amyloid polypeptide (amylin). In GDM, adipokines, such as leptin and adiponectin, are dysregulated and those might have both pathophysiological and prognostic significance in GDM.[6] Unbalanced maternal diet does not only results in immediate prenatal and postnatal adverse outcomes but also leads to long-term adverse consequences such as offspring's ability to challenge with unbalanced diet or physical inactivity in the future, i.e. insulin resistance and type 2 DM.[7] Although an association between thyroid antibodies and GDM has been proposed, this is significant but not strong.[8]

In pregnancy, metabolism is directed toward supplying enough nutrients to the growing fetus in form of amino acids and glucose. When there is shortage of these, free fatty acids, ketones, and glycerol may be used as maternal fuel. When compared to nonpregnant state, in overnight fasting, there is tendency for hypoglycemia and a greater rise in free fatty acids (i.e. accelerated starvation) in pregnancy and this is associated with hepatic insulin resistance. Parallel to the fetal placental unit growth in late pregnancy, there is decreased insulin sensitivity due to insulin resistance resulting from increased production of corticotropin-releasing hormone, growth hormone, human placental lactogen, and progesterone from the placenta. Tumor necrosis factor-alpha is also very important in the pathogenesis of insulin resistance. Although there is a physiologic insulin resistance in normal pregnancy, not all women develop GDM. GDM occurs when a woman's functional reserves of pancreas are not sufficient and she cannot produce larger amounts of insulin to overcome the insulin resistance. Those women are usually genetically predisposed to type 2 DM and may have suboptimal lifestyle. Patients who have a history of GDM have as high as 60% recurrence rate in the future pregnancies[9-11] and have approximately a 30% risk of developing DM type 2 within 10 years.[12,13]

Traditionally, GDM has been defined as onset or first recognition of abnormal glucose tolerance during pregnancy.[14,15] American College of Obstetricians and Gynecologists (ACOG) uses this terminology; however, the American Diabetes Association (ADA), the International Association of Diabetes and Pregnancy Study Groups (IADPSG), the World Health Organization (WHO), and the International Federation of Gynecology and Obstetrics (FIGO) use the term "gestational diabetes" to describe diabetes diagnosed rather during the second half of pregnancy in an attempt to distinguish pregestational diabetes first recognized during pregnancy from GDM[16-19] and use the terms "diabetes mellitus in pregnancy" or "overt diabetes" to describe diabetes which may be diagnosed by standard nonpregnant criteria early in pregnancy.

## EPIDEMIOLOGY

Gestational diabetes mellitus comprises approximately 87% of all diabetes in pregnancy, while pregestational diabetes mellitus (PDM) comprises the remaining 13%.[20] The prevalence of PDM has been increasing due to the increasing prevalence of type 2 diabetes in women of reproductive age and to the reclassification of some women previously diagnosed with "gestational diabetes" as "overt diabetes".[21] The prevalence of GDM is also increasing parallel to the increase in the prevalence of obesity[22] which is characterized by proinflammatory and insulin resistant state. In a population, the prevalence of GDM reflects the prevalence of type 2 diabetes; accordingly, people living in ethnic populations with a higher prevalence of type 2 diabetes have higher risk of GDM.[23]

Although all nations, both rich and poor, are suffering the impact of the diabetes epidemic, the poor and disadvantaged are suffering the most.[24] A study from the UK estimated the frequency of type 2 DM to be 1 in 955 births (0.10%).[25] According to 2014 National Diabetes Statistics Report 9.3% of the USA population has diabetes and 27.8% of people with diabetes are undiagnosed.[26] In the USA, the GDM prevalence may be as high as 9.2%[27] (range 1–25%[28]) and varies significantly between ethnic groups, locations,[29] differences in screening practices, testing method, diagnostic criteria, and population characteristics of pregnant women. Because some GDM patients have undiagnosed type 2 diabetes before pregnancy, the awareness of type 2 diabetes, screening strategies and definition affects the observed prevalence of GDM in that population. Although four international conferences have been organized in order to develop a consensus for the definition for GDM, this has failed and makes it hard to compare prevalence's of countries.[23] Using the new International Association of Diabetes in Pregnancy Study Group (IADPSG) criteria, the global prevalence of hyperglycemia first detected in pregnancy has been estimated at 16.9%.[30]

## SIGNIFICANCE

Diabetes during pregnancy (pregestational and gestational) has been associated with many adverse outcomes:

- Spontaneous abortion
- Fetal anomalies
- Preterm labor
- Infections: Vaginitis, urinary tract infections, pyelonephritis, endometritis, and post-operative wound infection[31]
- Diabetic ketoacidosis, diabetic nephropathy, diabetic retinopathy, and diabetic neuro-pathy
- Polyhydramnios
- Preeclampsia
- Shoulder dystocia
- Macrosomia and large for gestational age infant
- Fetal organomegaly (hepatomegaly and cardiomegaly)
- Operative delivery
- Maternal and infant birth trauma
- Perinatal mortality
- Neonatal complications (hypoglycemia, hypocalcemia, hyperbilirubinemia, and poly-cythemia).

Hyperglycemia is the primary mediator of these adverse outcomes, therefore tight glycemic control before and during pregnancy improves outcomes and is the key for treatment success.[32-34] Although women with type 2 DM have milder hyperglycemia and shorter duration of the disease, they do not have better outcomes than women with type 1 DM in terms of perinatal outcomes.[35] Even more, women with type 2 DM may be older, more obese, have higher parity and may be less likely to prepare for pregnancy and achieve good glycemic control than those with type 1 DM.[36,37] There is a continuous relation between the adverse outcomes and blood glucose levels. Hyperglycemia and adverse pregnancy outcomes (HAPO) study clearly demonstrated that there is no clear cut off level that defines patients at increased risk for birth weight greater than the 90th percentile, cesarean delivery, fetal hyperinsulinemia, and clinical neonatal hypoglycemia.[17,38] Women with GDM also have an increased risk of developing DM in later life. This risk is almost 50% 22–28 years after index pregnancy.[39,40]

## RISK FACTORS

Any women may develop GDM but some women due to risk factors have greater risk. Risk factors for GDM include:
- Maternal age above 25 years
- Family history of diabetes
- High risk ethnic groups having higher prevalence of type 2 diabetes
- Personal history of impaired glucose tolerance or gestational diabetes in a previous pregnancy
- Body mass index (BMI) above 30 kg/m$^2$
- Significant weight gain in early adulthood and between pregnancies
- Excessive gestational weight gain
- Previous delivery of a baby above 4.1 kg
- Previous birth of an infant with congenital anomaly or unexplained perinatal loss
- Polycystic ovary syndrome
- Maternal birth weight above 4.1 kg or below 6 2.7 kg
- Metabolic syndrome
- Glycosuria at the first prenatal visit
- Current use of glucocorticoids
- Hypertension.

Women at low risk of gestational diabetes include:
- No high risk ethnic group
- No family history for DM
- Maternal age below 25 years
- Normal BMI
- No history of glucose intolerance or adverse pregnancy outcomes which may be associated with gestational diabetes.

In fact, this low risk group constitutes only 10% of the general obstetric population and accordingly this is the basis for universal screening rather than selective screening.

## SCREENING AND DIAGNOSIS

The purpose of screening and diagnosing DM and GDM is identifying women with diabetes who may benefit from appropriate therapy and decrease fetal and maternal morbidity. Usually, screening is performed with a glucose-containing beverage followed by blood glucose level measurement. Unfortunately, there is no universal screening protocol; organizations have different screening and diagnostic policies. The screening is most cost effective in populations having high prevalence of GDM and type 2 DM. The screening may be universal (every pregnant patient is screened) or selective. Universal screening is more practical and logical because:

- Almost 90% of pregnant population has at least one risk factor for GDM[41]
- No risk factor is found in 2.7–20% of women who are diagnosed with GDM.[42,43]

Universal screening is performed at 24–28 weeks of gestation by either two-step approach [first 50 g oral glucose challenge test (OGCT) and then if screen positive followed by 100-g oral glucose tolerance test (OGTT)] or one-step approach (75 g OGTT). If the patient has high risk for GDM or PDM, the screening may be performed at first prenatal visit.

The recommendations of international organizations for screening are:

- International Association of Diabetes in Pregnancy Study Group (IADPSG)[17]: 75 g OGTT (Table 2.1).
- *American College of Obstetricians and Gynecologists:*[45] Two-step approach. Glucose more than or equal to 135 mg/dL or more than or equal to 140 mg/dL at 50-g glucose challenge test is elevated. The lower threshold provides greater sensitivity, but would result in more false positives. The lower threshold should be preferred in populations having higher prevalence of gestational diabetes. When the result is higher than threshold, 100 g OGTT should be performed. Fasting, 1 hour, 2 hours, and 3 hours blood glucose levels are measured. A positive test is defined by elevated glucose concentrations at two or more time points. Either Carpenter and Coustan thresholds or National Diabetes Data Group thresholds can be used (Table 2.1).
- World Health Organization:[19] 75 g OGTT
- American Diabetes Association:[18] Three different approaches:
  1. 50 g glucose challenge test and then if screen positive followed by 100 g OGTT
  2. 75 g OGTT
  3. Standard nonpregnant DM screening:
     - Hemoglobin A1c above 6.5%
     - Fasting blood glucose above 126 mg/dL
     - Postprandial blood glucose above 200 mg/dL and presence of classical DM symptoms.

**Table 2.1:** Range of diagnostic criteria for gestational diabetes.[44]

| Method | Criteria | Fasting mg/dL | 1-hour mg/dL | 2-hour mg/dL | 3-hour mg/dL |
|---|---|---|---|---|---|
| Two step (100 g load) | NDDG | 105 | 190 | 165 | 145 |
| | Carpenter and Coustan | 95 | 180 | 155 | 140 |
| Two step (75 g load) | CDA | 95 | 191 | 160 | |
| One step (75 g load) | WHO | 92–125 | 180 | 153–199 | |
| | IADPSG | 92–125 | 180 | 153 | |

(NDDG: National Diabetes Data Group; CDA: Canadian Diabetes Association; WHO: World Health Organization; IADPSG: International Association of Diabetes and Pregnancy Study Groups)

If a pregnant patient's random blood glucose level is above 200 mg/dL or fasting blood glucose level is above 126 mg/dL or has classical DM symptoms such as polydipsia, polyuria or loss of weight with unknown cause, she may be diagnosed with overt diabetes.[18]

In our opinion, it is reasonable to use one-step approach with 75 g OGTT as a diagnostic test and accept one abnormal value for diagnosis. Thus we avoid a screening test and proceed directly with a diagnostic test. One-step with moderate level of glucose load is easily accepted by the women and cause no serious side effects. With this policy, we diagnose more women with gestational diabetes. Using such policy is not just effective for gestational diabetes but also for obesity in pregnancy.

## MANAGEMENT

Women with pregestational diabetes should be counseled about the potential effects of diabetes on maternal and fetal outcomes. Those who have other coexisting medical conditions need further evaluation, as their treatments may have to be modified. The key components of preconceptional diabetes management are: tight glycemic control, knowledge of diabetes self-care, and medical optimization of preexisting complications and comorbidities associated with diabetes. When the pregnancy is planned and maternal glycemic control is established, the risk of stillbirth, neonatal death, and congenital malformations is reduced.[46-50]

Glycemic control, nutritional support, weight control, exercise, folic acid supplementation, and medication management are essential components of management of PDM patients during pregnancy. Multidisciplinary approach by diabetic and obstetric clinics is essential and provides better maternal and fetal risk prediction.

There is no consensus for the optimal timing of delivery. NIH workshop[51] recommendations for timing of delivery for PDM include:
- If the diabetes is well controlled and there is no vascular disease, delivery should be considered at more than or equal to 39 gestational weeks
- For those with vascular disease, delivery should be considered at 37–39 weeks
- For those with poor glycemic control, delivery should be considered after 34 gestational weeks.

NICE (National Institute for Health and Care Excellence) 2015 diabetes guideline[52] recommendations include:
- Women with PDM and no other complications should have elective birth by labor induction or elective cesarean delivery between 37+0 weeks and 38+6 weeks of pregnancy
- If there are maternal, fetal or metabolic complications, consider elective birth before 37+0 weeks.

After delivery, women should be advised to monitor glucose levels carefully particularly while breastfeeding in order to prevent hypoglycemia. Women typically revert to their prepregnancy insulin levels after delivery.[53] Those women should be reminded the importance of contraception and pregnancy planning before hospital discharge.

For GDM, maintaining good glycemic control is the key intervention for reducing the frequency and/or severity of complications. As in PDM, glycemic control is the cornerstone of management of GDM. The first step is diet therapy and exercise. If glycemic control cannot maintain normoglycemia and glucose levels are above the following thresholds (ACOG and ADA criteria), pharmacologic therapy is initiated:

- Fasting glucose level above 95 mg/dL
- 1-hour postprandial glucose level above 140 mg/dL
- 2-hour postprandial glucose level above 120 mg/dL.

Pharmacologic therapy may be given in the form of insulin or oral hypoglycemic agents. Food and Drug Administration has not specifically approved the latter option for GDM treatment.

Women with GDM managed with diet (GDM type A1) should not be delivered before 39 gestational weeks if there are no other complications.[51] Recommendation for women with GDM and treated with insulin (GDM type A2) is induction of labor at 39 weeks of gestation.[54] NICE[52] 2015 diabetes guideline advises to give birth no later than 40[+6] weeks and if there are maternal or fetal complications advises birth before 40[+6] weeks.

Women with GDM should have a fasting glucose measurement or 75 g OGTT at 6–12 weeks postpartum in order to diagnose overt DM.[45] According to ADA, if the results are normal, it should be repeated in at least every 3 years.[55]

## REFERENCES

1. Kampmann U, Madsen LR, Skajaa GO, et al. Gestational diabetes: a clinical update. World J Diabetes. 2015;6:1065-72.
2. Maahs DM, West NA, Lawrence JM, et al. Epidemiology of type 1 diabetes. Endocrinol Metab Clin North Am. 2010;39:481-97.
3. Devendra D, Liu E, Eisenbarth GS. Type 1 diabetes: recent developments. BMJ. 2004;328:750-4.
4. Vermeulen I, Weets I, Asanghanwa M, et al. Registry. Contribution of antibodies against IA-2β and zinc transporter 8 to classification of diabetes diagnosed under 40 years of age. Diabetes Care. 2011;34:1760-5.
5. Chiang JL, Kirkman MS, Laffel LM, et al. Type 1 diabetes through the life span: a position statement of the American Diabetes Association. Diabetes Care. 2014;37:2034-54.
6. Al-Badri MR, Zantout MS, Azar ST. The role of adipokines in gestational diabetes mellitus. Ther Adv Endocrinol Metab. 2015;6:103-8.
7. Kanaka-Gantenbein C. Fetal origins of adult diabetes. Ann N Y Acad Sci. 2010;1205:99-105.
8. Yang Y, Li Q, Wang Q. Thyroid antibodies and gestational diabetes mellitus: a meta-analysis. Fertil Steril. 2015;104:665-671.e663.
9. Getahun D, Fassett MJ, Jacobsen SJ. Gestational diabetes: risk of recurrence in subsequent pregnancies. Am J Obstet Gynecol. 2010;203:467.e461-6.
10. MacNeill S, Dodds L, Hamilton DC, et al. Rates and risk factors for recurrence of gestational diabetes. Diabetes Care. 2001;24:659-62.
11. Moses RG. The recurrence rate of gestational diabetes in subsequent pregnancies. Diabetes Care. 1996;19:1348-50.
12. Kaaja RJ, Greer IA. Manifestations of chronic disease during pregnancy. JAMA. 2005;294:2751-57.
13. Kintiraki E, Goulis DG, Mameletzi S, et al. Large- and small-for-gestational-age neonates born by women with gestational diabetes mellitus diagnosed by the new IADPSG criteria: a case-control study of 289 patients and 1 108 controls. Exp Clin Endocrinol Diabetes. 2013;121:262-5.
14. Classification and diagnosis of diabetes mellitus and other categories of glucose intolerance. National Diabetes Data Group. Diabetes. 1979;28(12):1039-57.

15. Proceedings of the 4th International Workshop-Conference on Gestational Diabetes Mellitus. Chicago, Illinois, USA. 14-16 March 1997. Diabetes Care. 1998;21 Suppl 2:B1-167.
16. Hod M, Kapur A, Sacks DA, et al. The International Federation of Gynecology and Obstetrics (FIGO) Initiative on gestational diabetes mellitus: A pragmatic guide for diagnosis, management, and care. Int J Gynaecol Obstet. 2015;131 Suppl 3:S173-211.
17. Metzger BE, Gabbe SG, Persson B, et al. International Association of Diabetes and Pregnancy Study Groups Consensus Panel. International association of diabetes and pregnancy study groups recommendations on the diagnosis and classification of hyperglycemia in pregnancy. Diabetes Care. 2010;33:676-82.
18. American Diabetes Association. (12) Management of diabetes in pregnancy. Diabetes Care. 2015;38 Suppl:S77-79.
19. WHO. Diagnostic Criteria and Classification of Hyperglycaemia First Detected in Pregnancy. [online] Available from: http://apps.who.int/iris/bitstream/10665/85975/1/WHO_NMH_MND_13.2_eng.pdf?ua=1 [Accessed July 2017].
20. Wier LM, Burgess J, Elixhauser A. Hospitalizations Related to Diabetes in Pregnancy, 2008: Statistical Brief #102. Healthcare Cost and Utilization Project (HCUP) Statistical Briefs [Internet]. Rockville (MD): Agency for Healthcare Research and Quality (US); 2006-2010 Dec.
21. Shaw JE, Sicree RA, Zimmet PZ. Global estimates of the prevalence of diabetes for 2010 and 2030. Diabetes Res Clin Pract. 2010;87:4-14.
22. Flegal KM, Carroll MD, Ogden CL, et al. Prevalence and trends in obesity among US adults, 1999-2008. JAMA. 2010;303:235-41.
23. Hunt KJ, Schuller KL. The increasing prevalence of diabetes in pregnancy. Obstet Gynecol Clin North Am. 2007;34:173-199, vii.
24. International Diabetes Federation. IDF Diabetes Atlas, 6th edition. Brussels, Belgium: International Diabetes Federation, 2013. [online] Available from: https://www.idf.org/e-library/epidemiology-research/diabetes-atlas.html [Accessed July 2017].
25. Confidential Enquiry into Maternal and Child Health (CEMACH). Pregnancy in women with Type 1 and Type 2 diabetes in 2002–2003, England, Wales and Northern Ireland. London: CEMACH; 2005.
26. National Diabetes Statistics Report: Estimates of Diabetes and Its Burden in the United States, 2014.
27. DeSisto CL, Kim SY, Sharma AJ. Prevalence estimates of gestational diabetes mellitus in the United States, Pregnancy Risk Assessment Monitoring System (PRAMS), 2007-2010. Prev Chronic Dis. 2014;11:E104.
28. Hartling L, Dryden DM, Guthrie A, et al. Screening and diagnosing gestational diabetes mellitus. Evid Rep Technol Assess (Full Rep). 2012:1-327.
29. Ferrara A. Increasing prevalence of gestational diabetes mellitus: a public health perspective. Diabetes Care. 2007;30 Suppl 2:S141-6.
30. Guariguata L, Linnenkamp U, Beagley J, et al. Global estimates of the prevalence of hyperglycaemia in pregnancy. Diabetes Res Clin Pract. 2014;103:176-85.
31. Schneiderman EH. Gestational diabetes: an overview of a growing health concern for women. J Infus Nurs. 2010;33:48-54.
32. Kitzmiller JL, Wallerstein R, Correa A, et al. Preconception care for women with diabetes and prevention of major congenital malformations. Birth Defects Res A Clin Mol Teratol. 2010;88:791-803.
33. Tennant PW, Glinianaia SV, Bilous RW, et al. Pre-existing diabetes, maternal glycated haemoglobin, and the risks of fetal and infant death: a population-based study. Diabetologia. 2014;57:285-94.
34. Jensen DM, Korsholm L, Ovesen P, et al. Peri-conceptional A1C and risk of serious adverse pregnancy outcome in 933 women with type 1 diabetes. Diabetes Care. 2009;32:1046-8.
35. Balsells M, García-Patterson A, Gich I, et al. Maternal and fetal outcome in women with type 2 versus type 1 diabetes mellitus: a systematic review and metaanalysis. J Clin Endocrinol Metab. 2009;94:4284-91.

36. Hewapathirana NM, Murphy HR. Perinatal outcomes in type 2 diabetes. Curr Diab Rep. 2014;14:461.
37. Murphy HR, Roland JM, Skinner TC, et al. Effectiveness of a regional prepregnancy care program in women with type 1 and type 2 diabetes: benefits beyond glycemic control. Diabetes Care. 2010;33:2514-20.
38. Landon MB, Gabbe SG. Gestational diabetes mellitus. Obstet Gynecol. 2011;118:1379-93.
39. O'Sullivan JB. Body weight and subsequent diabetes mellitus. JAMA. 1982;248: 949-52.
40. England LJ, Dietz PM, Njoroge T, et al. Preventing type 2 diabetes: public health implications for women with a history of gestational diabetes mellitus. Am J Obstet Gynecol. 2009;200:365. e361-368.
41. Danilenko-Dixon DR, Van Winter JT, Nelson RL, et al. Universal versus selective gestational diabetes screening: application of 1997 American Diabetes Association recommendations. Am J Obstet Gynecol. 1999;181:798-802.
42. Chevalier N, Fénichel P, Giaume V, et al. Hiéronimus. Universal two-step screening strategy for gestational diabetes has weak relevance in French Mediterranean women: should we simplify the screening strategy for gestational diabetes in France? Diabetes Metab. 2011;37:419-25.
43. Avalos GE, Owens LA, Dunne F, et al. ATLANTIC DIP Collaborators. Applying current screening tools for gestational diabetes mellitus to a European population: is it time for change? Diabetes Care. 2013;36:3040-4.
44. Vandorsten JP, Dodson WC, Espeland MA, et al. NIH consensus development conference: diagnosing gestational diabetes mellitus. NIH Consens State Sci Statements. 2013;29:1-31.
45. Committee on Practice Bulletins—Obstetrics. Practice Bulletin No. 137: Gestational diabetes mellitus. Obstet Gynecol. 2013;122:406-16.
46. Ray JG, O'Brien TE, Chan WS. Preconception care and the risk of congenital anomalies in the offspring of women with diabetes mellitus: a meta-analysis. QJM. 2001;94:435-44.
47. Steel JM, Johnstone FD, Hepburn DA, et al. Can prepregnancy care of diabetic women reduce the risk of abnormal babies? BMJ. 1990;301:1070-4.
48. Pearson DW, Kernaghan D, Lee R, et al. Scottish Diabetes in Pregnancy Study Group. The relationship between pre-pregnancy care and early pregnancy loss, major congenital anomaly or perinatal death in type I diabetes mellitus. BJOG. 2007;114:104-7.
49. Evers IM, de Valk HW, Visser GH. Risk of complications of pregnancy in women with type 1 diabetes: nationwide prospective study in the Netherlands. BMJ. 2004;328:915.
50. Temple RC, Aldridge VJ, Murphy HR. Prepregnancy care and pregnancy outcomes in women with type 1 diabetes. Diabetes Care. 2006;29:1744-9.
51. Spong CY, Mercer BM, D'alton M, et al. Timing of indicated late-preterm and early-term birth. Obstet Gynecol. 2011;118:323-33.
52. NICE. Diabetes in pregnancy (update). 2015 [online] Available from: https://www.nice.org.uk/guidance/ng3/documents/diabetes-in-pregnancy-update-full-draft-guidance2 [Accessed July 2017].
53. Egan AM, Murphy HR, Dunne FP. The management of type 1 and type 2 diabetes in pregnancy. QJM. 2015;108:923-7.
54. Rosenstein MG, Cheng YW, Snowden JM, et al. The risk of stillbirth and infant death stratified by gestational age in women with gestational diabetes. Am J Obstet Gynecol. 2012;206:309.e301-7.
55. American Diabetes Association. Standards of medical care in diabetes—2011. Diabetes Care. 2011;34 Suppl 1:S11-61.

# Chapter 3

# Overview of the Role of Ultrasound in the Management of Diabetes in Pregnancy

*Badreldeen Ahmed, Justin Konje*

## INTRODUCTION

Diabetes mellitus (DM) is one of the most common noncommunicable diseases (NCD), with serious consequences. NCD kill over 36 million people worldwide each year, of this 36 million, over 1.3 million are attributable to DM.[1] The St Vincent Declaration working group (1989) set a target of achieving pregnancy outcome in diabetic women that approximate that of nonpregnant women. The St Vincent Declaration was seen as an ambitious goal at the time. However, a member of this group, Michiel Krans,[2] follows this famous declaration by stating that, diabetic patients with or without pregnancy are no longer seen as patients, but as person with a disease that had important personal and social consequences. DM does not only affect the fetus but has a serious effect on the expectant mother. Women who develop diabetes for the first time during pregnancy, i.e. gestational diabetes mellitus (GDM), are more likely to develop GDM in future pregnancy and also type 2 DM in later life.[3-6] These expectant mothers are at the addition risks of hypertension and metabolic syndrome is later life.[7-9] However, the main objective of this review article is to discuss the effect of DM on the fetus. How much ultrasound contributed to this success in the management will be explored in this review article.

## ROLE OF ULTRASOUND IN ESTIMATION OF FETAL WEIGHT

The fetal growth and fetal size in diabetic pregnancy is a major concern for perinatologists. Most if not all obstetricians rely on ultrasound to estimate fetal weight (EFW). Monitoring of fetal growth will not be possible without accurate dating. Crown-rump length is the most accurate method of estimation of gestational age. In diabetic pregnancy, even this most accurate parameter is being challenged.[10-12] In diabetic pregnancy and because of maternal hyperglycemia, the glucose will cross to the fetus and causes excessive insulin production in the fetus. This fetal hyperinsulinemia will act on insulin-dependent organs and will result in macrosomia. The accepted definition of macrosomia now is infant weight of 4,500 g or above. Macrosomia is a real worry in diabetic patient with subsequent increase of shoulder dystocia, brachial plexus injury, clavicular injury, and maternal birth trauma to the bladder, perineum, and anal sphincter.[13-19] The situation is even more complicated in diabetic pregnancy because of the fact that the fat in diabetic fetus is disproportionally distributed, with fat accumulating mainly in the upper body and shoulder resulting in a higher chance of birth trauma even if the weight is not that significantly big.[20,21]

## Biometric Measurements

Most fetal medicine specialist and obstetricians rely on ultrasound parameters to EFW that includes the measurements of head circumference, biparietal diameter, abdominal circumference, and femur length in different combination.[22,23] The measurement of fetal weight using such parameters is grossly inaccurate; EFW can be in error by as much as 900 g, when infant weight is compared to EFW.[24] This difference is even further enhanced in diabetic pregnancy.[24] These different formula for EFW lack accuracy and uniformity and the situation is complicated even further by the fact that the standard of ultrasound scanning is very different between different institutions in different country and even in the same institution between individuals. Another major issue in the dilemma of EFW is that none of the used parameters of EFW taking consideration soft tissue thickness.[25-27] DM affect the abdominal circumference more than biparietal diameter, head circumference, and the femur length. All insulin-dependent organs in the fetus will be affected by diabetes; the only exception to this is the fetal brain. Abdominal circumference is probably one of the most accurate of these parameters to assess fetal weight. When the abdominal circumference is greater than 90th centile, macrosomia is found to be present in approximately 80% of neonates.[28,29] This difficulty in the estimation of fetal weight persuaded investigators to look for alternative parameters to measure to enhance the accuracy of fetal weight estimation. These alternative parameters include parameters such as:

- Cheek to cheek measurement[30-32]
- Measurement of fetal liver length[33]
- Subcutaneous fat in the lateral abdominal wall, mid-thigh circumference
- A combination of three markers for macrosomia which includes fetal fat layer, width of interventricular septum, and abdominal circumference.[34]

   None of the above tests showed clinical usefulness and did not stand the test of time.

## ROLE OF 3D ULTRASOUND IN EFW IN DIABETIC PREGNANCY

All the standard formula for estimation of fetal weight does not take soft tissue thickness in their estimation of fetal weight with the exception of fetal abdominal circumference. One of the promising soft tissue parameters to EFW is limbs volume.[35] Deter et al.[36] did a longitudinal study on the thigh circumference growth in the normal fetus as early as 1987. However, a land mark paper by Lee et al. in 2009,[37] provided normal reference ranges for fractional limbs volume (arm and thigh, Figs. 3.1A to D) measured using 3D ultrasound, as the a marker for fetus nutritional status and as an additional parameters to assess fetal weight more accurately. He also showed in the same paper[37] that these measurements are reproducible. Below is a brief description of the technique of how to obtain fractional limb volume.

## Fractional Limb Volume: Technical Consideration

Acquisition should be done when the fetus is very quiet and it is done in sagittal view. When the limb is seen, whether a thigh or an arm, you need to adjust the volume angle. When you are sure that the fetus is really quiet, you can release acquisition trigger. The volume will then be obtained (Figs. 3.2 and 3.3). Each limb volume will be subdivided into five equidistant slices. Bring the pivot point exactly in the middle of the bone. Then, measure the limb volume. Go

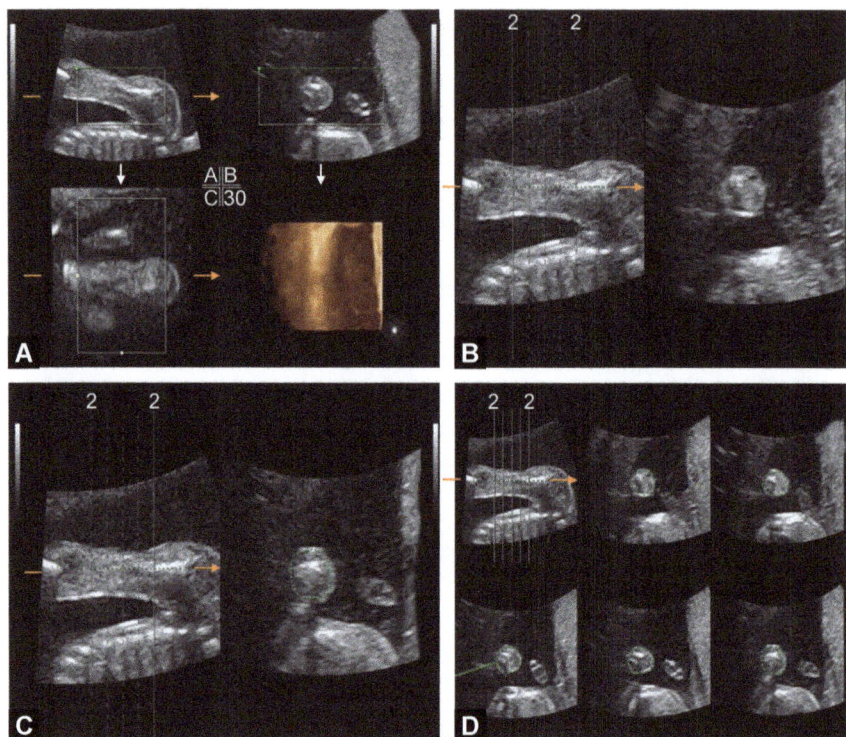

**Figs. 3.1A to D:** Fractional limb volume (hummers at 18 Weeks). In this view, the fetal arm is showed in the sagittal view, using the correct angel and when the fetus is quite. The vivid point is brought to the middle of the bone. (A) The caliber position is set at the beginning and the end of the arm; (B) Start calculation and you will then see a tomographic view of the arm; (C) Then you need to trace the fetal bone in five sections; (D) When you accept the region of interest, the result is the volume of the arm which can be used to modify the fetal weight.

to calculation, select fractional limb volume. The machine will give you two options, one for the arm and one for the thigh. Set the caliper position from the beginning to the end of the bone (femur or arm). Now, you will be having a tomographic view. You will trace the fetal bone in 5 sections, and you take it one by one, until you finish the five sections. Once the five sections has been traced and finished, you accept the volume. As the result, the volume of the thigh or the arm will appear which can be used for correction of fetal weight (Figs. 3.2A to D). We believe that such a technique can add accuracy to estimation of fetal weight and can be a clinically useful tool. However, it goes without saying these technique should only be used by the experienced trained operator with the right machine. Summary of the input of ultrasound in fetal weight estimation is given in Box 3.1.

## ROLE OF ULTRASOUND IN DIAGNOSIS OF CONGENITAL MALFORMATION

It is well established that the risk of fetal congenital malformation is much higher in GDM and pregestational diabetes mellitus (PGDM) compared to nondiabetic pregnant patients.

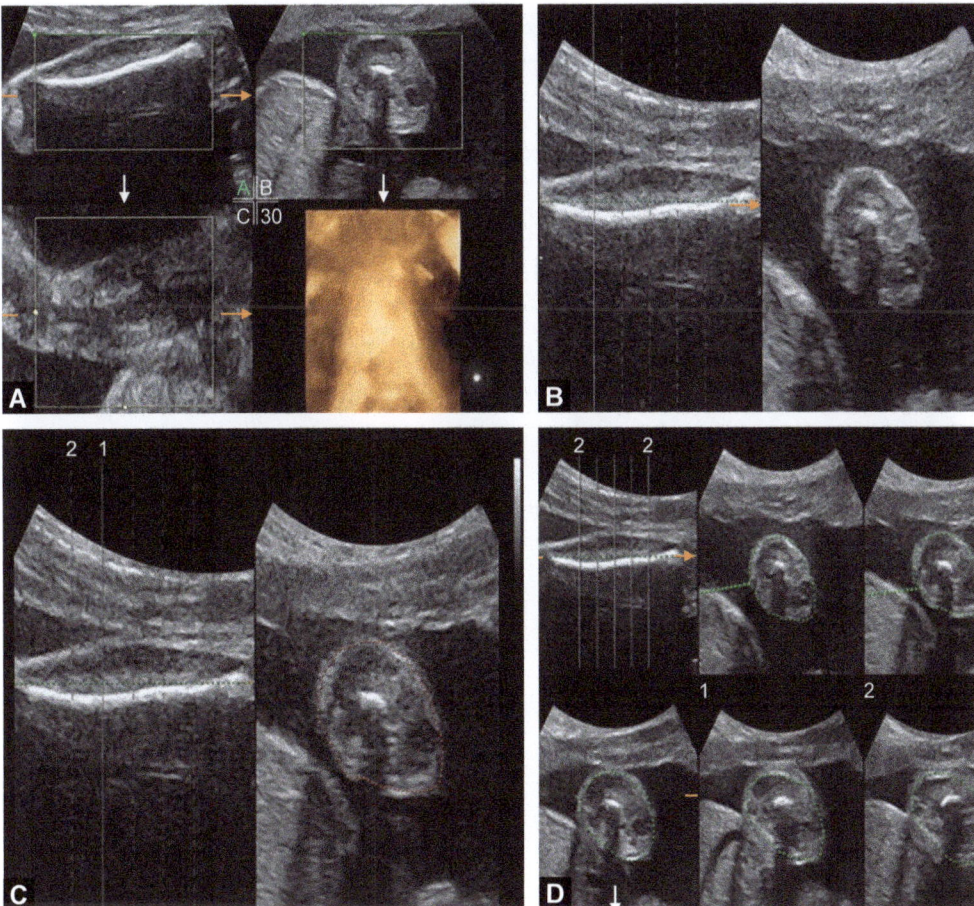

**Figs. 3.2A to D:** Fractional limb volume (thigh at 26 Weeks). In this view, the fetal femur is showed in the sagittal view, using the correct angel and when the fetus is quite. The vivid point is brought to the middle of the bone. (A) The caliber position is set at the beginning and the end of the femur; (B) Start calculation and you will then see a tomographic view of the thigh B; (C) Then you need to trace the fetal bone in five sections; (D) When you accept the region of interest, the result is the volume of the thigh which can be used to modify the fetal weight.

In most publications, the incidence of fetal malformations in this condition can be as high as 10%.[38-40] Fetal congenital malformation can affect virtually every single organ in the fetus in GDM and PGDM, however, this effect is more common in the central nervous system (CNS) and cardiovascular system. It was shown in many studies that about 50% of prenatal mortality in PGDM or GDM is attributable to congenital anomalies of which cardiac anomalies account for over 50%.[41-43]

## Central Nervous System

The CNS malformation encountered in PGDM and GDM include, anencephaly, spina bifida, microcephaly, and cranial regressions syndrome.[44-46] (Sacrococcygeal or lumbosacrococcygeal

> **Box 3.1:** Summary of the input of ultrasound in estimation of fetal weight.
> - The majority of general obstetricians and perinatologists rely on ultrasound in estimation of fetal weight
> - Ultrasound is not very accurate in estimation of fetal weight, regardless of the formulae used. The fact that the morphology of infant of diabetic mother is different from nondiabetic mother will only add to this inaccuracy
> - Compared to other ultrasound parameters used in estimation of fetal weight, fetal abdominal circumference is the most effective predictor of fetal weight
> - Fetal soft tissue parameters measured using ultrasound such as liver length, cheek to cheek, subcutaneous fat, and interventricular septum, did not gain any popularity and cannot be used for routine clinical work to estimate fetal weight
> - Fetal weight estimation using the new technique of fractional limb volume, which is a three-dimensional ultrasound, may improve detection and monitoring of fetus at risk of fetal growth deviation

agenesis accompanied by multiple skeletal anomalies). Much CNS malformation can be diagnosed by the end of the first trimester or beginning of second trimester with a very high degree of accuracy.[47-52] Complete and satisfactory visualization of central nervous malformation is best achieved during the anomaly scan 18–22 weeks of gestation. It is also possible to assess the CNS in late pregnancy; however, the views quality is reduced by calcified skull. A new approach is to use the MRI in selected CNS malformation to improve diagnostic accuracy of ultrasound. The use of MRI in such situations is only available in special centers and it not yet available a routine clinical practice.[53-56]

## Cardiovascular System

As mentioned earlier, fetal congenital anomalies are higher in GD and PGDM compared to nondiabetic pregnant patients. Congenital heart disease account for more than 50% of perinatal mortality and morbidity attributed to congenital fetal malformation.[57] Antenatal diagnosis of congenital heart disease improves prenatal outcome. It allows proper counseling of expecting parents and helps them be better prepared for the management and the outcome of their unborn fetus.[58] Diagnosis of congenital heart disease is not easy and it requires extensive training. Randall P performed a systematic review[59] which included five primary studies and concluded that the detection rate of congenital heart disease ranged between 35% and 86%. There are many reasons for this poor detection rate which include the heart is small and its size is changing with gestation, the heart is a moving organ and difficult to obtain all the right views and images, cardiac views are very much affected by the patient body mass index, and the presence or absence of scared tissues.[60]

The introduction of the concept of the four-chamber view for screening of the fetal heart was met with great expectations; however, several studies have showed that the performance of four-chamber view alone is very poor.[61,62] Chaoui R wrote a famous article for the Ultrasound Obstet Gynecol Journal entitled, the four-chamber view: four reasons why it seems to fail in screening for cardiac abnormalities and suggestions to improve detection rate.[63] In this article, he explained the reasons why the four-chamber view is not enough to diagnose congenital heart disease. He suggested that fetal echocardiography should routinely include the examination of the outflow tract mainly aorta from the left ventricles and pulmonary artery from the right ventricles and suggested that by doing so, the diagnostic accuracy of fetal echocardiography will improve significantly. However, even introduction of outflow tract examination does not seem to be enough and in a recent article written by DeVore et al.[64,65] found that only 13.7% of isolated congenital heart defect was detected during second trimester scan in over 92,000 screened pregnancies. For all the above mentioned reasons, any new diagnostic modalities are highly welcomed to improve antenatal detection of congenital heart disease.

Our first author in a review wrote an article entitled: The New 3D/4D based Spatio-temporal Imaging Correlation (STIC) in Fetal Echocardiography a promising tool for the future: published in previous issues of the Journal of Maternal Fetal Neonatal Med.[66] We will summarize her some important facts about this new modality.

## The New 3D/4D based Spatiotemporal Imaging Correlation (STIC) in Fetal Echocardiography

This technique relies on off-line volume analysis. The first and the most important step in this is to acquire an adequate volume. The volume is composed of a great number of two-dimension (2D) frames.[67] To acquire a good volume, you need to consider carefully the region of interest which determine the height and width of the volume, acquisition angle, and acquisition time and acquisition plan. The second step is volume analysis which can be presented using, multiplanar approach, tomographic ultrasound imaging or rendering.[61] Once volume analysis is complete we can move the region of interest across the cardiac views so we can move from the four-chamber view level (Fig. 3.3) to aorta outflow (Fig. 3.4) and then pulmonary artery and bifurcation (Fig. 3.5).[61] A new novel method called fetal intelligent navigation echocardiography was described recently by Yeol and Romero R for visualization of standard fetal echocardiography views from volume datasets obtained with STIC.[68] This new novel method can simplify examination of the fetal heart and reduce operator dependency. Summary of the input of ultrasound in diagnosis of congenital fetal malformation is given in Box 3.2.

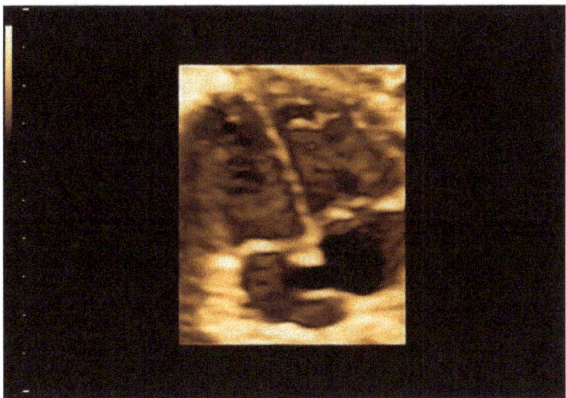

**Fig. 3.3:** This is a rendered 3D image of the heart obtained from the original heart volume. The image showing four-chamber view. This view gives a better prospective of the heart.

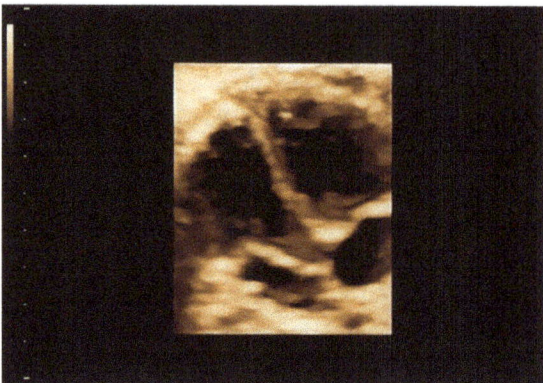

**Fig. 3.4:** This view demonstrates the left outflow tract. This view was obtained by moving the region of interest in Figures 3.6A to C toward the fetal head.

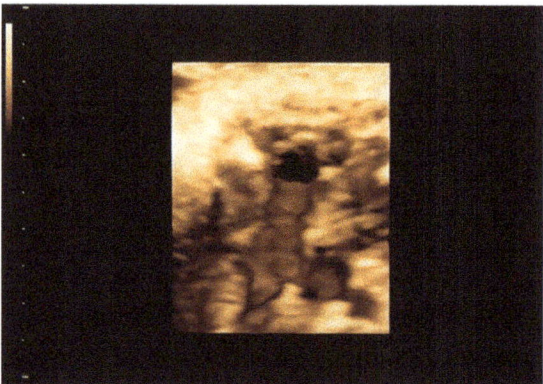

**Fig. 3.5:** This figure showed pulmonary artery dividing into two branches. This view is obtained by moving the region of interest further toward the fetal head.

---

**Box 3.2:** Summary of role of ultrasound in diagnosis of fetal congenital malformation.

- The risk of fetal congenital malformation is much higher in diabetic pregnancy compared to nondiabetic pregnant patients. In most publications, the incidence of fetal malformations in this condition can be as high as 10%
- Over 50% of perinatal mortality in diabetic pregnancy is attributable to fetal congenital malformation
- Fetal congenital malformation can affect virtually every single organ in the fetus in diabetic pregnancy; however, this effect is more common in the central nervous system (CNS) and cardiovascular system
- Virtually most of CNS malformation can be diagnosed by the end of the first trimester or beginning of second trimester with a very high degree of accuracy
- A new approach is to use the MRI in selected CNS malformation to improve diagnostic accuracy of ultrasound
- Diagnosis of congenital heart disease is not easy and it requires extensive training. The detection rate of congenital heart disease ranged between 35% and 86% and it remains a great challenge for perinatologists
- The New 3D/4D based Spatiotemporal Imaging Correlation (STIC) in Fetal Echocardiograph has the potential to improve detection of congenital cardiac defect. This technique relies on obtaining a volume from the moving fetal heart and off-line volume analysis

## ROLE OF ULTRASOUND IN MONITORING DIABETIC PREGNANT PATIENTS

It is well established that the prenatal morbidity and mortality are increased in diabetic pregnancy compared to nondiabetic pregnancies. There is an increased incidence of vascular consequences, hypertension, and preeclampsia in the mothers. Tight glucose control in these situations will improve the prenatal outcome.[69,70] Diabetic pregnancy will require proper fetal surveillance not only for the weight because of the risk of macrosomia but because of the added risk of fetal acidemia in diabetic pregnancy. Fetal acidemia caused by elevation in the fetal blood glucose level is an established concern in unexplained sudden intrauterine fetal death. Fetal hyperglycemia affects the fetus in many ways, first it causes an increase in the thromboxane/prostacyclin ratio in the umbilical vessels and in the placenta, and secondly it increases fetal hematocrit and polycythemia. Placental pathology in nondiabetic pregnancies has been successfully monitored and managed using Doppler flow in fetal vessel such as the umbilical artery and middle cerebral artery. The question is can we transfer Doppler criteria in these vessels to monitor the fetus in Diabetic pregnancy. Many authors believe that we cannot transfer Doppler criteria derived from conventional placental insufficiency cases to those in which diabetes is the main cause of metabolic changes involving soft tissue over growth, major metabolic changes, and a different vascular diameter.[71] Doppler studies in fetal vessels such as Umbilical artery and middle cerebral artery which perform brilliantly in identifying placental insufficiency in nondiabetic pregnancy, are not and neither appropriate nor sufficient in diabetic pregnancy.[71] The question remains of which vessels to interrogate in diabetic pregnancy. Ductus venosus (DV) has a promising potential identifying adverse perinatal outcome in such circumstances.[72] The fetal liver is another potential site to explore. The fetal liver plays a major metabolic role in intrauterine fetal life. The fetal liver growth is directly affected in diabetic pregnancy and it is a well-known fact that the increased in the abdominal diameter is mainly attributed to the large liver size. The liver growth is directly related to the blood flow in the umbilical vein.[73,74] Fetal liver perfusion is a very complex phenomena involving many vessels which include umbilical vein, DV, portal vein, and the hepatic artery.[75,76] The question is can we interrogate successfully vessels like DV,[71] fetal hepatic artery, and fetal portal system.[77] The Doppler studies in these vessels are a real challenge and require great degree of training and experience, not only that but to obtain an optimal result it needs to be done on a regular basis with a proper auditing mechanism in place. We will give a short account below of how to do Doppler blood flow in the DV and fetal hepatic artery.

## Ductus Venosus

Ductus venosus is a shunt between the umbilical vein and the inferior vena cava (IVC) that directs well-oxygenated blood through foramen ovale. This thin shunt is characterized by high blood velocity.[78] The changes in the DV blood velocity are reflection of the difference in the pressure gradient between the umbilical vein and the IVC which changed with different phase of cardiac cycle. Recording of DV Doppler is not easy and require special training and attention to many details.[79] Strict criteria need to be followed to optimize the results from DV blood flow studies, the further given practical points should be observed.

- Recording of the DV blood flow should be done when the fetus is quite. If the fetus is lying on its back, the best insonation will be on the midsagittal view through fetal abdomen, an alternative view will fetal oblige transverse abdominal view (Fig. 3.6A)
- The use of color Doppler is essential in identifying these minute vessels. The probe should be in line with blood flow in DV. Color Doppler setting should be very carefully adjusted to meet the requirement for proper recording. Theses adjustment include pulse repetition frequency (PRF), base line, velocity limit, and sample volume (Fig. 3.6B). To identify the high velocity within DV, the operator should use high PRF of 5–7 kHz, or velocity limit of 80–100 cm/s, a sample volume typically between 2 mm and 5 mm, and 0 angle of insonation
- The recorded waves should be of even appearance (Fig. 3.6C). The pulsatility index (PI) can be calculated automatically or manually. We then document absent or reversed a-wave velocity.[80,81]

## Fetal Hepatic Artery

The liver blood flow comes from the umbilical vein (70%), portal vein (20%), and hepatic artery (10%). Liver is the 4th preferential organ besides brain, heart, and the adrenals to be spared in hypovolemic or hypoxemic conditions.[82] Under physiological conditions, 80% of umbilical venous blood in the human fetus is distributed to the liver. The rest is shunted through DV.[83] Hypoxia causes release of catecholamine which dilate the ductus and divert more blood to the fetal heart at the expense of fetal liver. The liver produces adenosine which acts directly on the hepatic artery to cause dilation.

Measurement techniques and reference ranges for hepatic artery velocities and PI were established.[84] To optimize result when assessing hepatic artery Doppler:
The following criteria need to be applied (Fig. 3.7):
- Horizontal midsagittal view, magnify (only fetal trunk)
- Reduce gain, color map with small box
- Gate size (start 2 mm, measure 1 mm), insonation angle below 30°
- Filter 120 Hz, pulse width PRF 2.2–3.3 Hz.

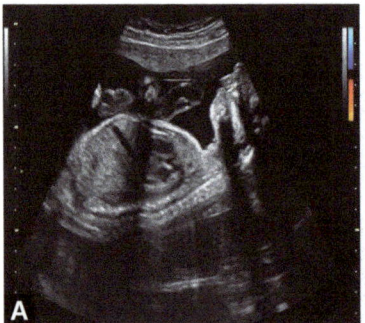
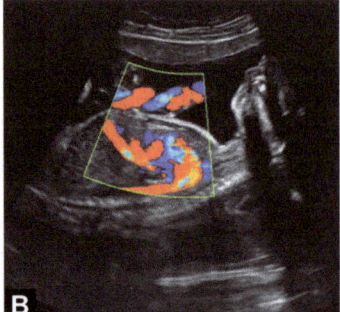
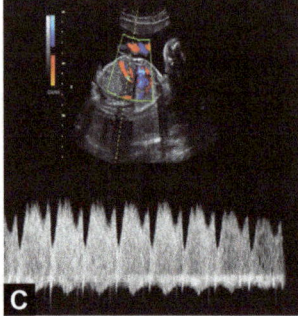

**Figs. 3.6A to C:** Ultrasound image showing correct insonation of the ductus venosus (DV) in sagittal view. (A) Recording of the DV blood flow should be done when the fetus is quite; (B) The use of color Doppler is essential in identifying these minute vessels; (C) The recorded waves should be of even appearance.

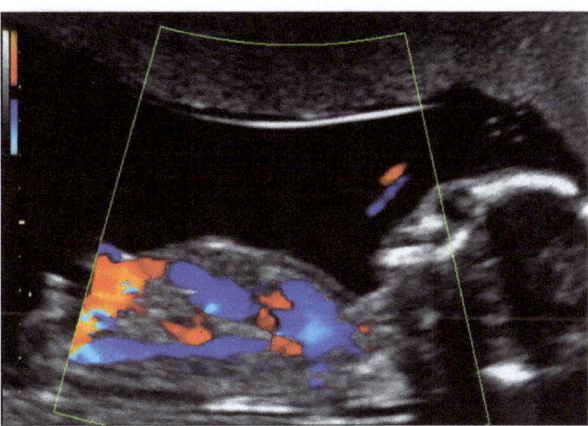

Fig. 3.7: Hepatic artery Doppler—steps and technique: Horizontal midsagittal view, magnify (only fetal trunk); Reduce gain, color map with small box; Gate size (start 2 mm, measure 1 mm), insonation angle <30°; Filter 120 Hz, pulse width pulse repetition frequency 2.2–3.3 Hz.

**Box 3.3:** Summary of the role of ultrasound in monitoring diabetic pregnant patients.

- Doppler studies in fetal vessels such as umbilical artery and middle cerebral artery which perform brilliantly in identifying placental insufficiency in nondiabetic pregnancy, are neither appropriate nor sufficient in diabetic pregnancy
- Ductus venosus (DV) has a promising potential identifying adverse perinatal outcome in diabetic pregnancy. However, recording of DV Doppler is not easy and requires special training and attention to many details. Strict criteria need to be followed to optimize the results from DV blood flow studies
- The fetal liver plays a major metabolic role in intrauterine fetal life. Fetal liver perfusion is a very complex phenomenon involving many vessels which include umbilical vein, Ductus venosus, portal vein, and the hepatic artery
- Hypoxia causes release of catecholamine which dilate the ductus and divert more blood to the fetal heart at the expense of fetal liver. The liver produces adenosine which acts directly on the hepatic artery to cause dilation. These changes make the hepatic artery a potential site to monitor the fetus in the diabetic pregnancy

In this review, we have discussed the established role of ultrasound in the management of pregnancy complicated by DM. We have also discussed some relatively new developments with regard to the use of ultrasound in this situation. Some of the techniques mentioned in this review are quite promising although not well established to be used in everyday practice and we want to emphasize the fact that such techniques should not be adopted without thorough training and continuous auditing.

Summary of the input of ultrasound in monitoring diabetic pregnant patients is given in Box 3.3.

## REFERENCES

1.  Lim SS, Vos T, Flaxman AD, et al. A comparative risk assessment of burden of disease and injury attributable to 67 risk factors and risk factor clusters in 21 regions, 1990-2010: a systematic analysis for the Global Burden of Disease Study 2010. Lancet. 2012;380(9859):2224-60.
2.  Michael Hall and Anne-Marie Felton (St) June 2009. Diabetes voice, Volume 54, Issue 2: 1-2. The St Vincent Declaration 20 years on – defeating diabetes in the 21st century.
3.  MacNeill S, Dodds L, Hamilton DC, et al. Rates and risk factors for recurrence of gestational diabetes. Diabetes Care. 2001;24:659-62.
4.  Moses RG. The recurrence rate of gestational diabetes in subsequent pregnancies. Diabetes Care. 1996;19:1348-50.
5.  Kjos SL, Buchanan TA, Greenspoon JS, et al. Gestational diabetes mellitus: the prevalence of glucose intolerance and diabetes mellitus in the first two months post partum. Am J Obstet Gynecol. 1990;163:93-9.
6.  Conway D, Langer O. Effects of new criteria for type 2 diabetes on the rate of postpartum glucose intolerance in women with gestational diabetes. Am J Obstet Gynecol. 1999;181:610-4.
7.  Reece EA. The fetal and maternal consequences of gestational diabetes mellitus. J Matern Fetal Neonatal Med. 2010;23:199-203.
8.  Vambergue A, Dognin C, Boulogne A, et al. Increasing incidence of abnormal glucose tolerance in women with prior abnormal glucose tolerance during pregnancy: DIAGEST 2 study. Diabet Med. 2008;25:58-64.
9.  Perkins JM, Dunn JP, Jagasia SM. Perspectives in gestational diabetes mellitus: a review of screening, diagnosis, and treatment. Clin Diabetes. 2007;25:57-62.
10. Pedersen JF, Molsted-Pederson L. Early growth delay retardation in diabetic pregnancy. BMJ. 1979;1:18.
11. Cousins L, Keys TC, Schorzman L, et al. Ultrasonographic assessment of early fetal growth in insulin-treated diabetic pregnancies. Am J Obstet Gynecol. 1988;159:1186.
12. Brown ZA, Mills JL, Metzger BE, et al. Early sonographic evaluation for fetal growth delay and congenital malformations in pregnancies complicated by insulin-requiring diabetes. National Institute of Child Health and Human Development Diabetes in Early Pregnancy Study. Diabetes Care. 1992;15:613-9.
13. Spellacy WN, Miller S, Winegar A, et al. Macrosomia-maternal characteristics and infant complications. Obstet Gynecol. 1985;66:158-61.
14. American College of Obstetricians and Gynecologists. Fetal macrosomia. ACOG Practice Bulletin No. 22. ACOG: Washington, DC, 2000.
15. Lipscomb KR, Gregory K, Shaw K. The outcome of macrosomic infants weighing at least 4500 g: Los Angeles County+University of Southern California experience. Obstet Gynecol. 1995;85:558-64.
16. Culligan PJ, Myers JA, Goldberg P, et al. Elective Caesarean section to prevent anal incontinence and brachial plexus injuries associated with macrosomia – a decision analysis. Int Urogynecol J. 2005;16:19-28.
17. Jolly MC, Sebire NJ, Harris JP, et al. Risk factors for macrosomia and its clinical consequences: a study of 350,311 pregnancies. Eur J Obstet Gynecol Reprod Biol. 2003;111:9-14.
18. Nesbitt TS, Gilbert WM, Herrchen B. Shoulder dystocia and associated risk factors with macrosomic infants born in California. Am J Obstet Gynecol. 1998;179:476-80.
19. Boney CM, Verma A, Tucker R, et al. Metabolic syndrome in childhood: association with birth weight, maternal obesity, and gestational diabetes mellitus. Pediatrics. 2005;115:e290-6.
20. Gilbert WM, Nesbitt TS, Danielsen B. Associated factors in 1611 cases of branchial plexus injury. Obstet Gynecol. 1999;93:536-40.
21. Roberts SW, Hernandez C, Maberry MC, et al. Obstetric clavicular fracture: the enigma of normal birth. Obstet Gynecol. 1995;86:978-81.

22. Landon MB, Gabbe SG, Sachs L. Management of diabetes mellitus and pregnancy: a survey of obstetricians and maternal–fetal specialists. Obstet Gynecol. 1990;75:635-40.
23. Hadlock FP, Harrist RB, Carpenter RJ. Sonographic estimation of fetal weight. The value of femur length in addition to head and abdomen measurements. Radiology. 1984;150:535-40.
24. Benson CB, Doubilet PM, Saltzman DH. Sonographic determination of fetal weights in diabetic pregnancies. Am J Obstet Gynecol. 1987;156:441-4.
25. Deter RL, Nazar R, Milner LL. Modified neonatal growth assessment score: a multivariate approach to the detection of intrauterine growth retardation in the neonate. Ultrasound Obstet Gynecol. 1995;6:400-10.
26. Vintzileos AM, Campbell WA, Rodis JF, et al. Fetal weight estimation formulas with head, abdominal, femur and thigh circumference measurements. Am J Obstet Gynecol. 1987;157:410-14.
27. MacLean F, Usher R. Measurements of liveborn fetal malnutrition infants compared with similar gestation and with similar birth weight normal controls. Biol Neonate. 1970;16:215-21.
28. Gilby JR, Williams MC, Spellacy WN. Fetal abdominal circumference measurements of 35 and 38 cm as predictors of macrosomia. J Reprod Med. 2000;45:936-8.
29. Tamura RK, Sabbagha RE, Depp R, et al. Diabetic macrosomia: accuracy of third trimester ultrasound. Obstet Gynecol. 1986;67:828.
30. Abramowicz JS, Sherer DM, Woods JR. Ultrasonographic measurement of cheek-to-cheek diameter in fetal growth disturbances. Am J Obstet Gynecol. 1993;169:405-8.
31. Abramowicz JS, Robischon K, Cox C. Incorporating sonographic cheek-to-check diameter, biparietal diameter and abdominal circumference improves weight estimation in the macrosomic fetus. Ultrasound Obstet Gynecol. 1997;9:409-13.
32. Abramowicz JS, Sarosh R, Abramowicz S. Fetal cheek-to-cheek diameter in the prediction of mode of delivery. Am J Obstet Gynecol. 2005;192:1205-13.
33. Roberts AB, Mitchell J, Murphy C, et al. Fetal liver length in diabetic pregnancy. Am J Obstet Gynecol. 1994;170:1308-12.
34. Bethune M, Belli R. Evaluation of the measurement of the fetal fat layer, interventricular septum and abdominal circumference percentile in the prediction of macrosomia in pregnancies affected by gestational diabetes. Ultrasound Obstet Gynecol. 2003;22:586-90.
35. Jeanty P, Romero R, Hobbins JC. Fetal limb volume: a new parameter to assess fetal growth and nutrition. J Ultrasound Med. 1985;4:273-82.
36. Deter RL, Rossavik IK, Cortissoz C, et al. Longitudinal studies of thigh circumference growth in normal fetuses. J Clin Ultrasound. 1987;15:388-93.
37. Lee W, Balasubramaniam M, Deter RL, et al. Fractional limb volume – a soft tissue parameter of fetal body composition: validation, technical considerations and normal ranges during pregnancy. Ultrasound Obstet Gynecol. 2009;33:427-40.
38. Mills JL, Knopp RH, Simpson JL, et al. Lack of relation of increased malformation rates in infants of diabetic mothers to glycemic control during organogenesis. N Engl J Med. 1988;318:671-6.
39. Shields LE, Gan EA, Murphy HF, et al. The prognostic value of hemoglobin A1c in predicting fetal heart disease in diabetic pregnancies. Obstet Gynecol. 1993;81:954-7.
40. Albert TJ, Landon MB, Wheller JJ, et al. Prenatal detection of fetal anomalies in pregnancies complicated by insulin-dependent diabetes mellitus. Am J Obstet Gynecol. 1996;174:1424-8.
41. Becerra JE, Khoury MJ, Cordero JF, et al. Diabetes mellitus during pregnancy and the risks for specific birth defects: a population-based controlled study. Pediatrics. 1990;85:1-9.
42. Kucera J. Rate and type of congenital anomalies among offspring of diabetic women. J Reprod Med. 1971;7:61-70.
43. Landon MB, Gabbe SG. Diabetes and pregnancy. Med Clin North Am. 1988;72:1493-511.
44. Twickler D, Budorick N, Pretorius D, et al. Caudal regression versus sirenomelia: sonographic clues. J Ultrasound Med. 1993;12:323-30.
45. Subtil D, Cosson M, Houfflin V, et al. Early detection of caudal regression syndrome: specific interest and findings in three cases. Eur J Obstet Gynecol Reprod Biol. 1998;80:109-112.

46. Zaw W, Stone DG. Caudal regression syndrome in twin pregnancy with type 2 diabetes. J Perinatol. 2002;22:171-4.

47. Ghi T, Pilu G, Savelli L, et al. Sonographic diagnosis of congenital anomalies during the first trimester. Placenta. 2003;24 (Suppl B):S84-S87.

48. Monteagudo A, Timor-Tritsch IE. First trimester anatomy scan: pushing the limits. What can we see now? Curr Opin Obstet Gynecol. 2003;15:131-41.

49. Bronshtein M, Ornoy A. Acrania: anencephaly resulting from secondary degeneration of a closed neural tube: two cases in the same family. J Clin Ultrasound. 1991;19:230-4.

50. Blaas HG, Eik-Nes SH, Vainio T, et al. Alobar holoprosencephaly at 9 weeks gestational age visualized by two- and three-dimensional ultrasound. Ultrasound Obstet Gynecol. 2000;15:62-5.

51. Blaas HG, Eik-Nes SH, Isaksen CV. The detection of spina bifida before 10 gestational weeks using two- and three-dimensional ultrasound. Ultrasound Obstet Gynecol. 2000;16:25-9.

52. Johnson SP, Sebire NJ, Snijders RJ, et al. Ultrasound screening for anencephaly at 10–14 weeks of gestation. Ultrasound Obstet Gynecol. 1997;9:14-16.

53. Levine D, Barnes PD, Robertson RR, et al. Fast MR imaging of fetal central nervous system abnormalities. Radiology. 2003;229:51-61.

54. Griffiths PD, Paley MN, Widjaja E, et al. In utero magnetic resonance imaging for brain and spinal abnormalities in fetuses. BMJ. 2005;331:562-5.

55. Malinger G, Ben-Sira L, Lev D, et al. Fetal brain imaging: a comparison between magnetic resonance imaging and dedicated neurosonography. Ultrasound Obstet Gynecol. 2004;23:333-40.

56. Malinger G, Lev D, Lerman-Sagie T. Is fetal magnetic resonance imaging superior to neurosonography for detection of brain anomalies? Ultrasound Obstet Gynecol. 2002;20:317-21.

57. Rosano A, Botto LD, Botting B, et al. Infant mortality and congenital anomalies from 1950 to 1994: an international perspective. J Epidemiol Community Health. 2000;54:660-6.

58. Chiappa E. The impact of prenatal diagnosis of congenital heart disease on pediatric cardiology and cardiac surgery. J Cardiovasc Med (Hagerstown). 2007;8(1):12-6.

59. Randall P, Brealey S, Hahn S, et al. Accuracy of fetal echocardiography in the routine detection of congenital heart disease among unselected and low risk populations: a systemic review. BJOG. 2005;112(1):24-30.

60. Devore GR, Falkensammer P, Sklansky MS, et al. Spatio-temporal image correlation (STIC): new technology for evaluation of the fetal heart. Ultrasound Obstet Gynecol. 2003;22:380-7.

61. Crane JP, LeFevre ML, Winborn RC, et al. Randomized trial of prenatal ultrasonographic screening: impact on the detection, management, and outcome of anomalous fetuses. The RADIUS Study Group. Am J Obstet Gynecol. 1994;171:392-9.

62. Stoll C, Alembic Y, Dott B, et al. Evaluation of prenatal diagnosis of congenital heart disease. Prenat Diagn. 1998;18:801-7.

63. Chaoui R. The four-chamber view: four reasons why it seems to fail in screening for cardiac abnormalities and suggestions to improve detection rate. Ultrasound Obstet Gynecol. 2003;22(1):3-10.

64. DeVore GR, Falkensammer P, Sklansky MS, et al. Spatio-temporal image correlation (STIC): new technology for evaluation of the fetal heart. Ultrasound Obstet Gynecol. 2003;22(4):380-7.

65. DeVore GR, Polanko B. Tomographic ultrasound imaging of the fetal heart: a new technique for identifying normal and abnormal cardiac anatomy. J Ultrasound Med. 2005;24(12):1685-96.

66. Ahmed B. The new 3D/4D based spatio-temporal imaging correlation (STIC) in fetal echocardiography: a promising tool for the future. J Matern Fetal Neonatal Med. 2014;27(11):1163-8.

67. DeVore GR, Falkensammer P, Sklansky MS, et al. Spatio-temporal image correlation (STIC): new technology for evaluation of the fetal heart. Ultrasound Obstet Gynecol. 2003;22(4):380-7.

68. Yeo L, Romero R. Fetal Intelligent Navigation Echocardiography (FINE): a novel method for rapid, simple, and automatic examination of the fetal heart. Ultrasound Obstet Gynecol. 2013;42(3):268-84.

69. Gabbe SG, Graves CR. Management of diabetes mellitus complicating pregnancy. Obstet Gynecol. 2003;102:857-68.

70. Stuart A, Amer-Wahlin I, Gudmundsson S, et al. Ductus venosus blood flow velocity waveform in diabetic pregnancies. Ultrasound Obstet Gynecol. 2010;36:344-9.
71. Kiserud T. Diabetes in pregnancy: scanning the wrong horizon? Ultrasound Obstet Gynecol. 2010;36:266-7.
72. Wong SF, Petersen SG, Idris N, et al. Ductus venosus velocimetry in monitoring pregnancy in women with pregestational diabetes mellitus. Ultrasound Obstet Gynecol. 2010;36(3):350-4.
73. Pietryga M, Brazert J, Wender-Ozegowska E, et al. Abnormal uterine Doppler is related to vasculopathy in pregestational diabetes mellitus. Circulation. 2005;112:2496-500.
74. Tchirikov M, Kertschanska S, Schroder HJ. Obstruction of ductus venosus stimulates cell proliferation in organs of fetal sheep. Placenta. 2001;22:24-31.
75. Tchirikov M, Kertschanska S, Sturenberg HJ, et al. Liver blood perfusion as a possible instrument for fetal growth regulation. Placenta. 2002;23:S153-8.
76. Haugen G, Hanson M, Kiserud T, et al. Fetal liver-sparing cardiovascular adaptations linked to mother's slimness and diet. Circ Res. 2005;96:12-4.
77. Kessler J, Rasmussen S, Godfrey K, et al. Longitudinal study of umbilical and portal venous blood flow to the fetal liver: low pregnancy weight gain is associated with preferential supply to the fetal left liver lobe. Pediatr Res. 2008;63:315-20.
78. Kiserud T, Eik-Nes SH, Blaas HG, et al. Ultrasonographic velocimetry of the fetal ductus venosus. Lancet. 1991;338:1412-4.
79. Maiz N, Kagan KO, Milovanovic Z, et al. Learning curve for Doppler assessment of ductus venosus flow at 11 + 0 to 13 + 6 weeks' gestation. Ultrasound Obstet Gynecol. 2008;31:503-6.
80. Hecher K, Campbell S, Snijders R, et al. Reference ranges for fetal venous and atrioventricular blood flow parameters. Ultrasound Obstet Gynecol. 1994;4:381-90.
81. Kessler J, Rasmussen S, Hanson M, et al. Longitudinal reference ranges for ductus venosus flow velocities and waveform indices. Ultrasound Obstet Gynecol. 2006;28:890-8.
82. Kiserud T. Blood flow and the degree of shunting through the ductus venosus in the human fetus. Am J Obstet Gynecol. 2000;182 (1 Pt 1):147-53.
83. Kilavuz O. Is the liver of the fetus the 4th preferential organ for arterial blood supply besides brain, heart, and adrenal glands. J Perinat Med. 1999;27(2):103-6.
84. Ebbing C, Rasmussen S, Godfrey K, et al. Hepatic artery hemodynamics suggest operation of a buffer response in the human fetus. Reprod Sci. 2008;15:166-78.

# Chapter 4

# Fetal Behavior in Normal Pregnancy and Diabetic Pregnancy

*Asim Kurjak, Sonal Panchal*

## INTRODUCTION

Ultrasound has been a modality of choice for assessment of the development of the embryo and fetus in the womb. Three-dimensional (3D) ultrasound has made the study of the fetal anatomy even more accurate and understandable. But the fetal development is not only the development of the structures, it is also their functionality. The functionality of the kidneys, for example can be confirmed by urine production and filling of the bladder, the functionality of the bladder by its periodically emptying and filling and that of the heart by fetal circulation. The function of the nervous system is the most complex and this can be studied by fetal movements and fetal expressions. The development of fetal motor behaviors can be studied by real-time ultrasound.[1] The fetal activity observed or recorded with ultrasound equipment is fetal behavior.[2]

Study of the fetal movements has been found to be more correlating with the fetal central nervous system (CNS) development. Studies have shown that the development and maturation of the fetal nervous system is reflected by quality and quantity of fetal movements.[3,4] On comparing the fetal movements with morphological studies, it was found that the fetal behavioral patterns directly reflected the development and maturation of fetal CNS. Therefore, assessment of fetal behavior in different periods of gestation can help to distinguish normal brain from abnormal during different phases of development.[5] It also helps to make the diagnosis of functional and structural abnormalities earlier.[6]

B-mode or a two-dimensional (2D) ultrasound is impossible to understand the complexity of these movements and so till the invent of four-dimensional (4D) ultrasound it was not possible to correctly evaluate the fetal movements, especially fetal expressions. The details of fetal face and hands studied by 4D ultrasound have potential to generate information regarding fetal movement and behavior.[7] There is a specific fetal behavioral pattern that corresponds to each week or trimester of fetal life and this pattern reflects the steps of human brain development and maturation.[8-10]

## UNDERSTANDING THE NORMAL FETAL ACTIVITY

Spontaneous fetal movements can be observed using 2D ultrasound around 8th of gestational week, but 4D ultrasound may show fetal motility at 7th week of gestation on transvaginal scans.[11,12] From 10 weeks onwards the frequency of fetal movements increase and are maximum between 14 weeks and 19 weeks.[12] The longest interval between movements at this age is 5–6 minutes. Between 9 weeks and 14 weeks of fetal age mostly general movements are observed.[13]

Using 4D sonography, Kurjak et al. found that from 13 gestational weeks onwards, a "goal orientation" of hand movements (Figs. 4.1A to C) appears and a target point can be recognized for each hand movement. At 15 weeks, 15 different types of movements have been recorded.[14,15] But according to a study by Kurjak et al., 16 different types of movements can be observed at 15 weeks of gestation.[16] Eye movements are detectable at 16–18 weeks, organized complex movements at 20 weeks and facial expressions also start at 20 weeks.[17] Facial expressions like smiling, yawning, eyelid movement, mouthing, grimacing, tongue expulsion/swallowing, and sucking were observed during 2nd and 3rd trimesters. Mouthing was the most frequent facial movement during early 3rd trimester, whereas scowling and sucking were the least frequent.[15-18] In the second half of pregnancy, the frequency of general movements gradually decreases, particularly during the last 10 weeks of pregnancy.[19] In the last trimester of gestation, the range of hand and face movements is the widest.[19] Fetal neuromuscular development is due to alternate periods of increased and decreased movements, though the exact functional significance of the same is still not understood.[20,21]

The movement in an unstimulated fetus is the result of spontaneous behavior without sensory stimulation and is the best method to assess its CNS capacity,[5] and can be used as a marker for fetal brain status.[22] Any fetal brain insult will interfere with endogenous motor activity of the fetus. Genetic factors, external stimuli, pathological conditions or even environmental changes, can affect the fetal human brain up to a degree that may be difficult to assess, especially prenatally. Most times the neurological damage and its effects are difficult to predict.[23]

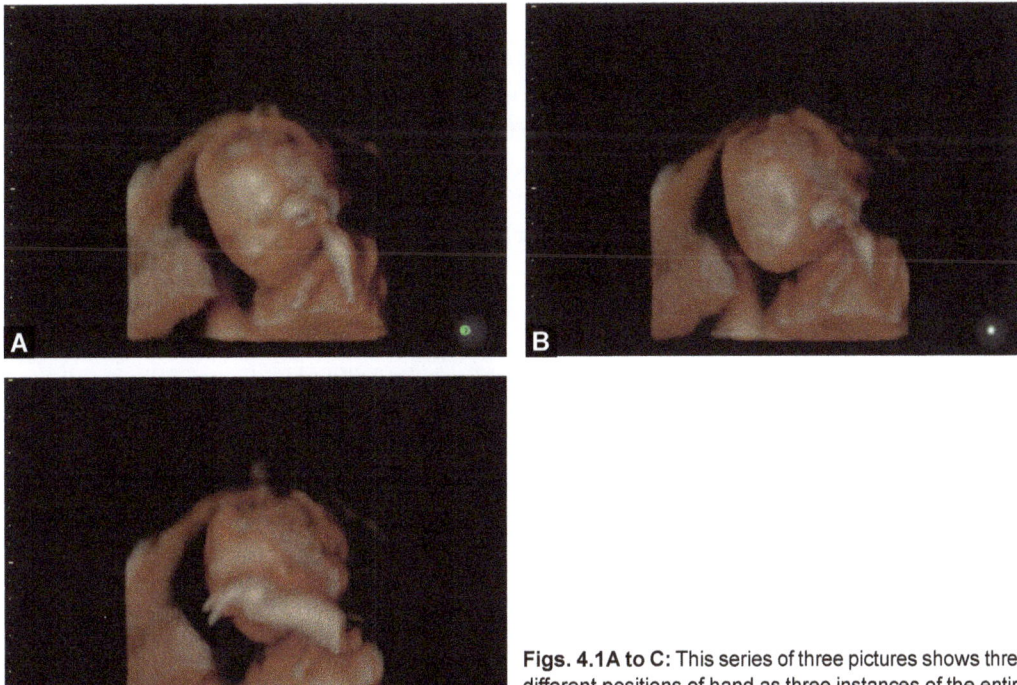

**Figs. 4.1A to C:** This series of three pictures shows three different positions of hand as three instances of the entire movement of hand to face.

| Table 4.1: Types of hand and facial movements in fetus.[28] | |
|---|---|
| *Hand and head movements* | *Facial expression* |
| • Head retroflexion<br>• Head rotation<br>• Head anteflexion<br>• Hand to head direction<br>• Hand to eye<br>• Hand to mouth<br>• Hand to face<br>• Hand to ear | • Isolated eye blinking<br>• Mouthing<br>• Yawning<br>• Tongue expulsion<br>• Grimacing<br>• Swallowing |

Establishment of neural connections as a developmental process leads to development of new movement patterns of fetus or transformation of existing patterns.[24]

Integrity of the fetal CNS can be assessed by behavioral states of the fetus viz. movement of individual organs like head, trunk or limbs in an unstimulated but awake fetus and also by qualitative assessment of general movements.[25] When fetal behavior is studied by 4D ultrasound, the altered movement pattern can diagnose abnormal brain development and assist early diagnosis of various abnormalities.[26-28]

The centers in the cerebellum impose controls on the unrestricted movements induced by the lower centers of the brain.[19] The movements also become more complex as pregnancy advances that represents the cerebral maturation. Inhibition is a marker of neurological development (especially cortical centers) and most longitudinal studies have also proved that the fetus becomes less active as gestation advances.[29]

Movements observed and analyzed in 2nd and 3rd trimesters are listed in Table 4.1.

The spinothalamic tract is established at the 20th week and myelinized by 29 weeks of gestation and the thalamocortical connections penetrate the cortical plate at 24–26 weeks.[16] Evoked potentials can be detected from the cortex at the 29th week, indicating that the functional connection between periphery and cortex operates from that time onwards.[30,31] This is because of maturation process in the brainstem.[32] Facial expressions are representation of the maturation of the brain. Expressions like grimacing, tongue expulsion and eyelid movements (Figs. 4.2A and B) similar to emotional expressions in adults and can be seen by 4D US.[17]

General movements (GMs) or Gestalt perception[33] involve the whole body in a variable sequence of arm, leg, neck, and trunk movements. The movements increase and decrease in intensity, but are fluent and elegant, complex, and variable. These are called fetal or preterm from 28 to 36 to 38 weeks of postmenstrual age. GMs are considered to be a better predictor of postnatal neurological disability than clinical neurological examination alone.[33]

Normal GMs are complex but fluent and involve neck, trunk, and limb movements. Moreover these should also increase and decrease in their intensity.[34] GMs are complex and fluent and also are not repetitive.[35] If that is not the case, they are considered abnormal.[15,35] Slow, monotonous repetitive movements mimicking cramps are abnormal movements. Even when the movements are occurring with generalized simultaneous muscle contractions and relaxations, it is considered abnormal pattern.[5,22] These also may show variability in strength and the amplitude of movements.[22] These are often seen in the fetuses of mothers with diabetes

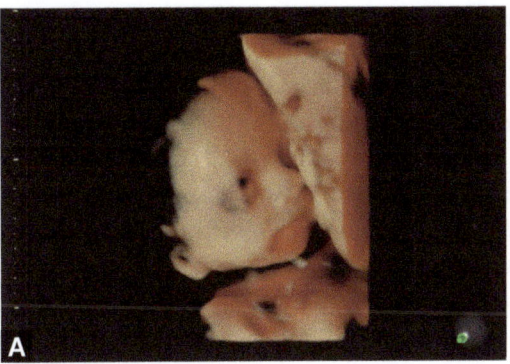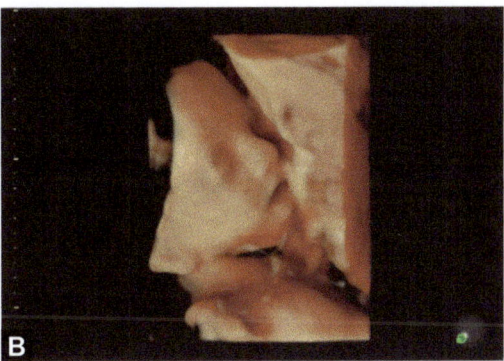

**Figs. 4.2A and B:** (A and B) Eyelid and lip movements are seen. (A) The eye is open and mouth is closed and (B) Eye is closed and the mouth is open in the same fetus.

mellitus, and also other pregnancies at risk like intrauterine growth retardation (IUGR), pregnancy-induced hypertension (PIH), and prematurity.[15] Both term and preterm newborns, who had cerebral insult of any type during their prenatal period may also show abnormal general movement.[11] The identification of fetal CNS depression is based on precompetences (opening of eyes, variety of facial expressions) also along with the primary reflexes (rhythmical bursts in the sucking pattern) and quality of GMs.[5,36]

Evaluation of GMs must be done on video recordings, may it be prenatal or postnatal. These must be evaluated with "Gestalt perception", which could be described as overall impression of GMs with standardized procedure. It is important to recognize, document and classify the movement pattern and then their complexity, variability, and fluency.[23] These can be classified as normal-optimal, normal-suboptimal, mildly abnormal, and definitely abnormal.[5,37] Quality of neurological movement is more important than the quantity. These can better predict neurodevelopmental outcome than classical neurologic examination alone.[38]

## Why do Fetuses of Diabetic Mothers have Higher Risk of Neurological Derangements?

Gestational diabetes mellitus, with it carries multiple risk factors for the developing fetus, and each have independent effects on neurodevelopment that may impact mnemonic behavior.[39] These risk factors are: (1) chronic hypoxia,[40] (2) hyperglycemia/reactive hypoglycemia, and (3) iron deficiency.[41] On the basis of animal models, these factors selectively affect regions of the fetal brain that are involved in explicit memory (e.g. the hippocampus).[39,42-44]

Women with diabetic vascular disease have the highest malformation rates, leading to the belief that vascular disease and hypoxia are teratogenic.[44]

Maternal ketonuria in diabetic mothers is associated with reduced intelligence quotient (IQ) in their infants,[44-46] as ketones may interfere with normal development of fetal brain.[44] Abnormal protein synthesis might also result from a lack of glucogenic amino acids or an overabundance of branched-chain amino acids as is seen in poorly controlled diabetes.[44,47] Jovanovic and co-workers (1980) were able to study the pregnancy in diabetic women before the 10th week of gestation. Women with uncontrolled diabetes had estradiol, prolactin, and human chorionic gonadotropin levels below the range associated with normal pregnancy.[44,48]

When these risk factors co-occur, oxygen consumption of the fetus increases and causes fetal hypoxia[39,49] that can ultimately result in brain iron deficiency through shifting of available fetal iron away from the brain and into the expanding red cell mass.[39,41] Prenatal hypoxia and hyperglycemia/reactive hypoglycemia cause poor behavioral and neurologic outcomes presenting as motor and cognitive deficits in humans[41] and damage to memory areas such as the cerebral cortex, striatum, and hippocampus in animal models.[39,50] These factors together lead to altered normal maturation of the behavioral states in fetuses with IUGR, maternal diabetes mellitus or alcohol consumption.[51]

## What to Observe for?

### Assessment of Neurological Function

Even when these movements were documented by 4D ultrasound it was a very difficult task to classify these movements and based on these to judge the neurological developmental status of fetus. For the first time a test was structured to assess the fetal CNS integrity and was named as Kurjak's antenatal neurodevelopmental test (KANET).[52] KANET is the first test that is based on 4D ultrasound, with an original scoring system and has been standardized, so it can be implemented in everyday practice, overcoming the practical difficulties and covering the gaps of methods that were used in the past for the evaluation of fetal behavior (Table 4.2).[53-54] Improvement of 4D USG technology enabled introduction of KANET, which is a powerful tool in the assessment of fetal behavior and a guide to predict cerebral palsy.[55] After experimental use for 10 years, a consensus was passed in Bucharest concluding that KANET test can be used in everyday clinical practice for follow-up of fetuses at neurological risk with strong recommendations for strict and reliable multidisciplinary postnatal follow-up for at least 3 years. It has acceptable sensitivity, specificity, positive, and negative predictive value for neurodevelopmental anomalies.[56]

The test is of more significance than the morphological studies of the brain. Analysis of the fetal behavior compared with morphological studies has concluded that fetal behavioral patterns are direct reflection of developmental and maturational processes of fetal CNS.[57]

The parameters that have been incorporated in the KANET test are isolated head anteflexion, overlapping cranial sutures, head circumference, isolated eye blinking, facial alterations, mouth opening (yawning or mouthing), isolated hand and leg movements and thumb position, and Gestalt perception of GMs.[44,58]

Based on multicentric studies over several years, and on the theory of central pattern generators for GMs, certain fetal movements were chosen as parameters to assess neurological development.[58,59] It is to be performed between 28 weeks and 38 weeks, when fetus is awake. Fetus is observed for 15–20 minutes. If fetus is asleep, the scan is repeated after 30 minutes or after 14–16 hours. Each movement depending on its frequency is given a score of 0, 1, and 2 for nine parameters. A score of 0–5 is abnormal, a score of 6–13 is borderline and a score of more than 14 is normal.[60] If the test is abnormal or borderline, it is to be repeated every 2 weeks, till delivery.[59]

**Table 4.2:** Score chart of fetal movements according to KANETs.[62]

| Sign | Score 0 | Score 1 | Score 2 | Sign score |
|------|---------|---------|---------|------------|
| Isolated head anteflexion | Abrupt | Small range (0–3 times of movements) | Variable in full range, many alternation (>3 times of movements) | |
| Cranial sutures and head circumference | Overlapping of cranial sutures | Normal cranial sutures with measurement of HC below or above the normal limit (−2 SD) according to GA | Normal cranial sutures with normal measurement of HC according to GA | |
| Isolated eye blinking | Not present | Not fluent (1–5 times of blinking) | Fluency (>5 times of blinking) | |
| Facial alteration (grimace or tongue expulsion) Or Mouth opening (yawning or mouthing) | Not present | Not fluent (1–5 times of alteration) | Fluency (>5 times of alteration) | |
| Isolated leg movement | Cramped | Poor repertoire or Small in range (0–5 times of movement) | Variable in full range, many alternation (>5 times of movements) | |
| Isolated hand movement Or Hand to face movements | Cramped or abrupt | Poor repertoire or Small in range (0–5 times of movement) | Variable in full range, many alternation (>5 times of movements) | |
| Fingers movements | Unilateral or bilateral clenched fist, (neurological thumb) | Cramped invariable finger movements | Smooth and complex, variable finger movements | |
| Gestalt perception of GMs | Definitely abnormal | Borderline | Normal | |
| | | | **Total score** | |

(GA: Gestational age; GMs: General movements; HC: Head circumference; KANETs: Kurjak's antenatal neurodevelopmental tests).

## Neurological Function in Fetus of a Diabetic Female

The results of a study by Edelberg et al. (1987) and Robertson et al. have shown that it is actually the changing maternal blood glucose level that affects the cyclicity and frequency of fetal motor activity, rather than persistently high blood glucose levels.[21,61,70]

Schulte et al. and Visser et al.[62,80] studied the neurological development of infants of diabetic mothers, and found longer rapid eye movement (REM) sleep in newborn infants of diabetic mothers.

There is evidence that it is the concurrent maternal blood glucose levels according to which the fetal movements may be affected in diabetic and nondiabetic pregnancies, but different studies have mixed results. Some studies have reported increased and some have shown decreased fetal movement with elevated blood glucose levels.[21,63-68]

Some have reported decreased fetal movement,[69-71] and others have reported no effects.[72-76] An increased rate of minor neurological dysfunction was found in a group of 32 children born to mothers with gestational diabetes, including some fine and gross motor deficits, compared with a group of control children.[77,78]

Abnormalities in the fetal motor activity may consist of a delayed first emergence of specific movements, quantitative changes and an abnormal quality of movements (i.e. changes in execution of movement patterns) and abnormal development of fetal behavioral states.[50,56,57] Qualitative and quantitative assessment of fetal movements can be used for the recognition of cerebral dysfunctions and probably neuromuscular ailments. Alteration in the normal movement pattern in terms of frequency and strength is seen in IUGR, the pathophysiology of which is fetal hypoxia. In the fetuses of diabetic mothers, fetal hypoxia is the main pathophysiological factor and so similar changes in fetal movements can be observed. A study on diabetes-related influence on fetal motor activity revealed 1–2 week delayed appearance of almost all fetal behavioral patterns in first 12 weeks of pregnancy except the fetal breathing movements.[15,50]

Fetal breathing pattern is considered to be one of the important parameters of fetal well-being in late diabetic pregnancies. It is not affected by Braxton–Hicks contractions. This means that the fetal neural control of fetal breathing like movements differ in diabetic pregnancy, than in normal.[15,79]

## Cyclic Motility

Other aspects of fetal neurobehavioral organization are influenced by the altered metabolic environment.[70,80-90] In spite of good clinical control of diabetes, the infants of these mothers have a risk of compromised neurological developmental outcome.[21,91-99]

Spontaneous fetal movement in the last trimester of human gestation is dominated by irregular oscillations on a scale of minutes [cyclic motility (CM)].[21] The movement pattern (increased and decreased movements in cyclicity in normal females) is steady but is altered in mothers with increased blood glucose levels.[21] Early in the 3rd trimester, changes in the rate of oscillation in fetal CM between the two periods of activity were inversely related to changes in maternal blood glucose levels.[21] It is seen that relatively short-term fluctuations in maternal glucose metabolism, rather than chronically elevated blood glucose, per se, is the effective perturbation of the intrinsic cyclic patterns in spontaneous fetal motor activity in diabetic pregnancies. The results revealed that fetal CM is more sensitive to fluctuations in maternal blood glucose levels during the early part of the 3rd trimester of gestation than during the middle or end of the 3rd trimester. The results suggest that disruption of the temporal organization of spontaneous fetal motor activity in diabetic pregnancies represents an acute response to fluctuations in the metabolic environment rather than alteration of CM development.[100,101]

But according to other studies, the transient abnormality maternal glucose metabolism may affect fetal CM but does not cause any increased risk of poor general developmental outcome in children of diabetic mothers.[21,100] The effects are similar in the fetuses of mothers with type I or gestational diabetes, and no difference when fetuses later classified as appropriate for large gestational age were considered separately (p > 0.05).[21,100]

## Effect during Infancy and Childhood

When gross motor functions were studied in children of diabetic mothers by the Bruininks-Oseretsky test of motor proficiency, it was observed that these children were weak performers as compared to the controls.[77] Maternal diabetes adversely affects some fine neurological functions in children at school age, but not their cognitive scores.[77] These effects are not correlated with the degree of glycemic control.[77] Developmental delay, learning difficulties at school, and a high rate of attention deficit hyperactivity disorders (ADHDs) are more often seen in the children born after high-risk pregnancies.[77,102] These children in their early school age have more soft neurological signs (signs of mild, nonspecific brain damage), and lower gross and fine motor achievements than pair matched control children born to nondiabetic mothers.[77,103,104] Variability in muscle tone (hypertonicity or hypotonicity) may cause delayed or abnormal motor development (Miyahara M, Department of Kinesiology, UCLA; unpublished observations).

Children born to the mothers having diabetes mellitus (IDM) had a risk of shorter gestational age [mean 38 weeks, standard deviation (SD) 2], greater standardized birth weight scores (mean 3,797 grams, SD 947), and lower iron stores (mean ferritin concentration 87 µg/L, SD 68) in comparison with the control group.[39]

Children born to the mothers whose diabetes was diagnosed late in pregnancy, had lower cognitive scores and verbal performance compared with controls.[77,105,106]

## Can KANET Predict these Abnormalities?

Kurjak's antenatal neurodevelopmental test can be useful for early diagnosis of neurological disorders that become manifest in perinatal and postnatal period.[46] The authors observed that a low KANET score is predictive of both intrauterine or neonatal death.[53] The study demonstrated the evaluated and accepted KANET to detect and discriminate normal and abnormal fetal behavior in normal and in high-risk pregnancies.[107] Except for higher incidence in the abnormal group, there was no marked difference in the different motor patterns studied.[108,109]

Analysis of sick preterm infants revealed a "reduction of elegance" and fluency, variability, fluctuation in intensity, and speed instead of change in incidence of distinct motor patterns.[30,110-112] Abo-Yaqoub et al. showed in their study that the difference between the two groups were isolated head anteflexion (Figs. 4.3A to C), isolated eye blinking, facial expressions, mouth movements (Figs. 4.4A to C), finger movements (Figs. 4.5A to C), isolated hand movements, hand-to-face movements (Figs. 4.6A to C), and GMs (Figs. 4.7A to D). For isolated leg movements (Figs. 4.8A and B), and cranial sutures, the difference was not significant.[113]

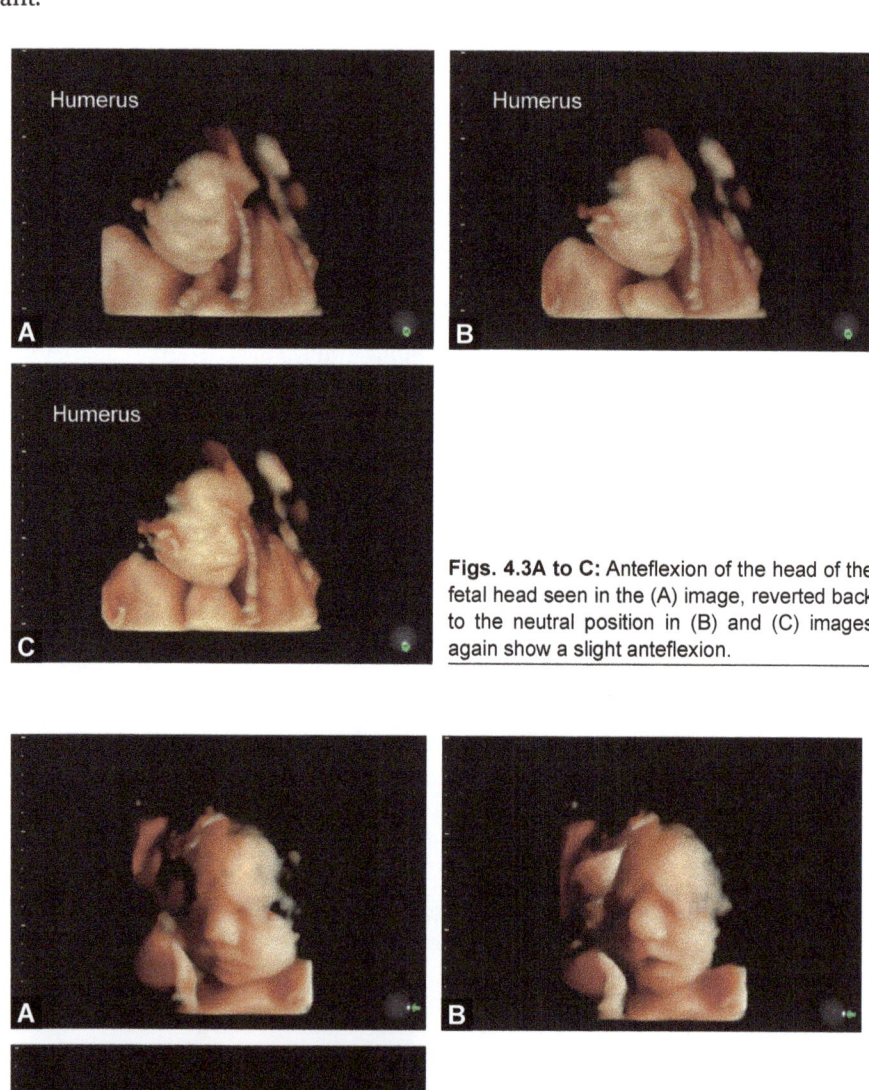

**Figs. 4.3A to C:** Anteflexion of the head of the fetal head seen in the (A) image, reverted back to the neutral position in (B) and (C) images again show a slight anteflexion.

**Figs. 4.4A to C:** The series of images from (A) to (C) shows opening of the fetal mouth.

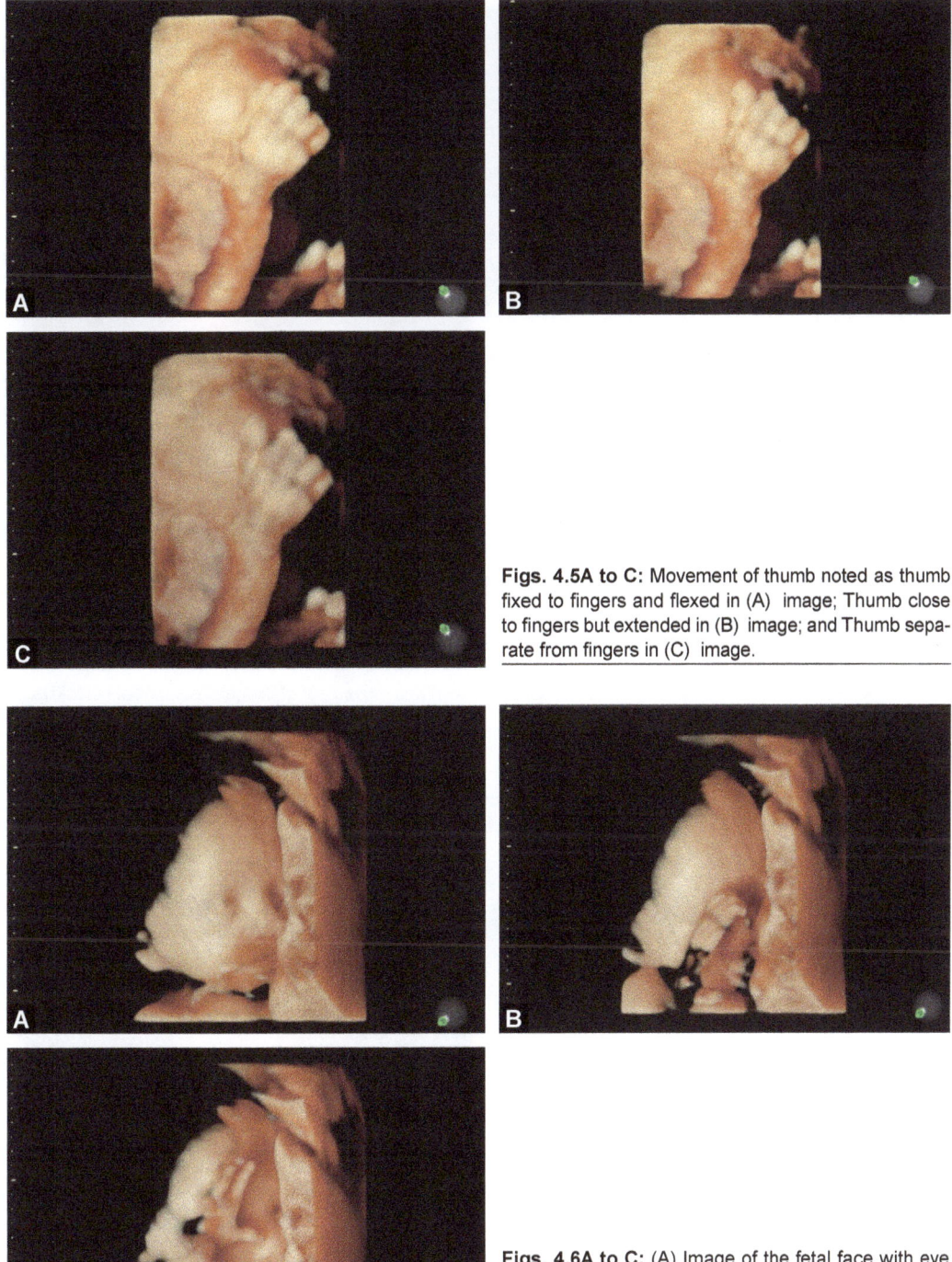

**Figs. 4.5A to C:** Movement of thumb noted as thumb fixed to fingers and flexed in (A) image; Thumb close to fingers but extended in (B) image; and Thumb separate from fingers in (C) image.

**Figs. 4.6A to C:** (A) Image of the fetal face with eye open and hand close to the chin; (B) The hand raised to fetal eye and eye is hidden by the hand; and (C) Supination of the hand and abduction of thumb and extension of fingers.

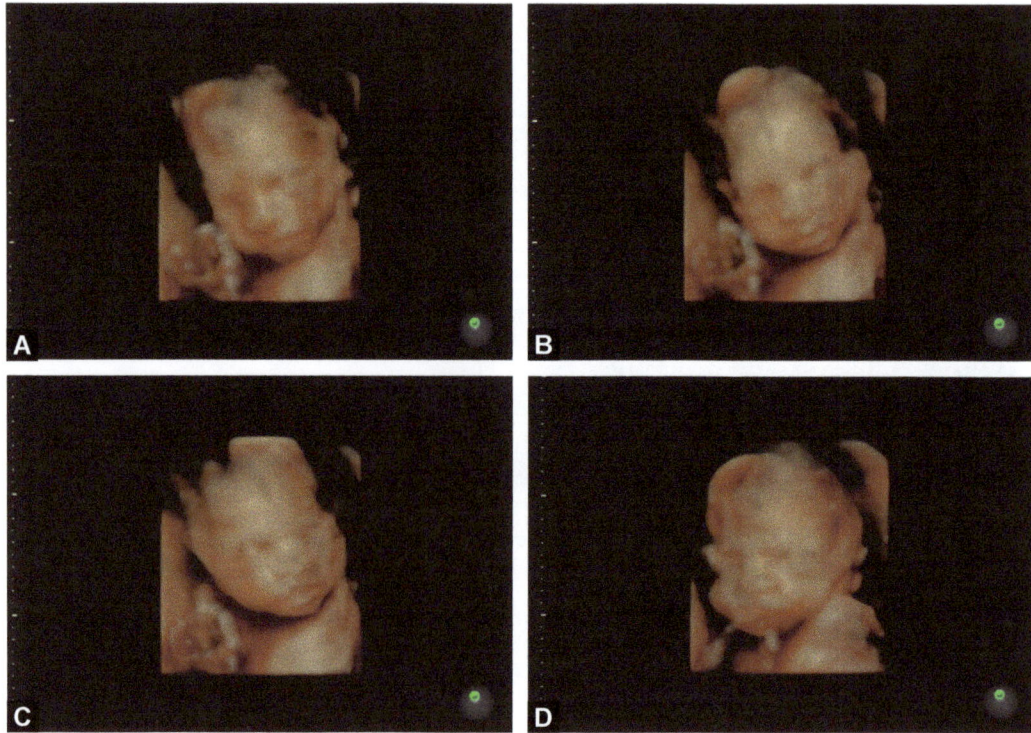

**Figs. 4.7A to D:** Fetal head rotation and anteflexion movement with movement of the hand seen from (A) to (D), as a part of general movement.

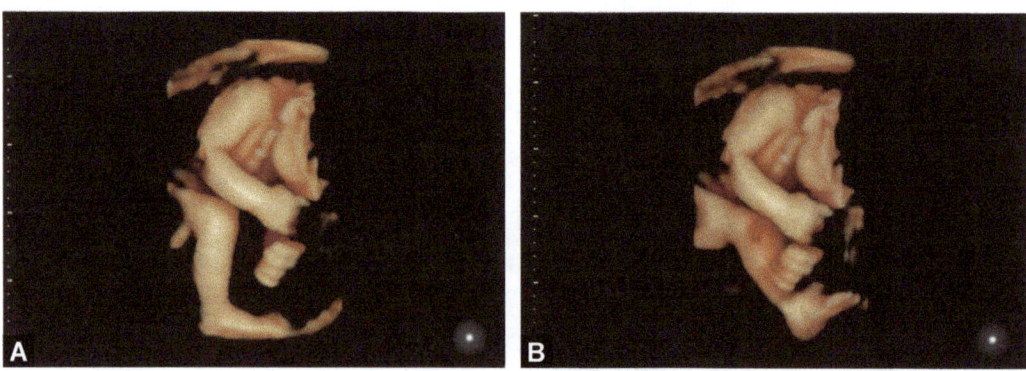

**Figs. 4.8A and B:** (A) Partially flexed leg is seen and (B) Extension of the same is seen.

Athanasiadis et al., in 2013, applied KANET test to assess and compare fetal behavior and neurodevelopment in 152 pregnant women, classified as low-risk (n = 78) and high-risk (n = 74) pregnancies in the 2nd and 3rd trimester.[39] The neurodevelopmental score was statistically significantly higher in the low-risk group compared to the high-risk group.[39] Though the score was higher in diabetes subgroup compared to the IUGR and the preeclampsia subgroup.[113]

## CONCLUSION

Inadequate glycemic control and vascular pathologies are the chief causes of neurological developmental inadequacies in fetuses of diabetic mothers. These can be assessed and predicted antenatally by KANET test.

## REFERENCES

1. Roodenburg PJ, Wladimiroff JW, van Es A, et al. Classification and quantitative aspects of fetal movements during the second half of normal pregnancy. Early Hum Dev. 1991;25(1):19-35.
2. de Vries JI, Fong BF. Normal fetal motility: an overview. Ultrasound Obstet Gynecol. 2006;27(6): 701-11.
3. Prechtl HF. Qualitative changes of spontaneous movements in fetus and preterm infant are a marker of neurological dysfunction. Early Hum Dev. 1990;23(3):151-8.
4. DiPietro JA. Neurobehavioral assessment before birth. Ment Retard Dev Disabil Res Rev. 2005;11(1):4-13.
5. Kurjak A, Predojevic M, Stanojevic M, et al. Intrauterine growth restriction and cerebral palsy. Acta Inform Med. 2010;18(2):64-82.
6. Einspieler C, Prechtl HF, Ferrari F, et al. The qualitative assessment of general movements in preterm, term and young infants—review of the methodology. Early Hum Dev. 1997;50(1):47-60.
7. Moster D, Wilcox AJ, Vollset SE, et al. Cerebral palsy among term and postterm births. JAMA. 2010;304(9):976-82.
8. Yigiter AB, Kavak ZN. Normal standards of fetal behavior assessed by four-dimensional sonography. J Matern Fetal Neonatal Med. 2006;19(11):707-21.
9. Rees S, Harding R. Brain development during fetal life: influences of the intra-uterine environment. Neurosci Lett. 2004;361(1-3):111-4.
10. Kurjak A, Carrera JM, Stanojevic M, et al. The role of 4D sonography in the neurological assessment of early human development. Ultrasound Rev Obstet Gynecol. 2004;4(3):148-59.
11. Araki M, Nishitani S, Ushimaru K, et al. Fetal response to induced maternal emotions. J Physiol Sci. 2010;60(3):213-20.
12. Salihagić-Kadić A, Medić M, Kurjak A, et al. Four-dimensional sonography in the assessment of fetal functional neurodevelopment and behavioral patterns. Ultrasound Rev Obstet Gynecol. 2005;5(2):154-68.
13. Andonotopo W, Kurjak A, Azumendi G. Ultrasound studies on early pregnancy. In: Carrere JM, Kurjak A (Eds). Atlas of Clinical Application of Ultrasound in Obstetrics and Gynecology, 1st edition. New Delhi: Jaypee Brothers Medical Publishers (P) Ltd; 2006.
14. Azumendi G, Arenas JB, Andonotopo W, et al. Three-dimensional sonoembryology. In: Kurjak A, Arenas JB (Eds). Donald School Textbook of Transvaginal Sonography, 1st edition. New Delhi: Jaypee Brothers Medical Publishers (P) Ltd; 2006.
15. Kurjak A, Predojevic M, Stanojevic M, et al. The use of 4D imaging in the behavioral assessment of high risk fetuses. Imaging Med. 2011;3(5):557-69.
16. Kurjak A, Carrera J, Medic M, et al. The antenatal development of fetal behavioral patterns assessed by four-dimensional sonography. J Matern Fetal Neonatal Med. 2005;17(6):401-16.
17. Andonotopo W, Medic M, Salihagic-Kadic A, et al. The assessment of fetal behavior in early pregnancy: comparison between 2D and 4D sonographic scanning. J Perinat Med. 2005;33(5): 406-14.
18. de Vries JI, Visser GH, Prechtl HF. The emergence of fetal behavior. I. Qualitative aspects. Early Hum Dev. 1982;7(4):301-22.
19. D'Elia A, Pighetti M, Moccia G, et al. Spontaneous motor activity in normal fetuses. Early Hum Dev. 2001;65(2):139-47.

20. Kurjak A, Stanojevic M, Andonotopo W, et al. Behavioral pattern continuity from prenatal to post-natal life—a study by four-dimensional (4D) ultrasonography. J Perinat Med. 2004;32(4):346-53.
21. Robertson SS, Dierker LJ. Fetal cyclic motor activity in diabetic pregnancies: sensitivity to maternal blood glucose. Dev Psychobiol. 2003;42(1):9-16.
22. Einspieler C, Prechtl HF, Bos A, et al. Prechtl's Method on the Qualitative Assessment of General Movements in Preterm, Term and Young Infants, 1st edition. Cambridge: Mac Keith Press; 2008.
23. Yan F, Dai SY, Akther N, et al. Four-dimensional sonographic assessment of fetal facial expression early in the third trimester. Int J Gynecol Obstet. 2006;94(2):108-13.
24. Robertson SS. Mechanism and function of cyclicity in spontaneous movement. In: Smotherman WP, Robinson SR (Eds). Behavior of the Fetus. Caldwell: Telford Press; 1989. pp. 77-94.
25. Nijhuis JG. Fetal Behavior, Developmental and Perinatal Aspects. Oxford: Oxford University Press; 1992.
26. Kurjak A, Luetic AT. Fetal neurobehavior assessed by three-dimensional/four-dimensional sonography. Zdrav Vestn. 2010;79:790-9.
27. Amiel-Tison C, Gosselin J, Kurjak A. Neurosonography in the second half of fetal life: a neonatologist's point of view. J Perinat Med. 2006;34(6):437-46.
28. Kurjak A, Azumendi G, Vecek N, et al. Fetal hand movements and facial expression in normal pregnancy studied by four-dimensional sonography. J Perinat Med. 2003;31(6):496-508.
29. Ten Hof J, Nijhuis IJ, Mulder EJ, et al. Longitudinal study of fetal body movements: nomograms, intrafetal consistency, and relationship with episodes of heart rate patterns A and B. Pediatr Res. 2002;52(4):568-75.
30. Kurjak A, Andonotopo W, Stanojevic M, et al. Longitudinal study of fetal behavior by four-dimensional sonography. Ultrasound Rev Obstet Gynecol. 2005;5(4):259-74.
31. Kostovic I, Rakic P. Development of prestriate visual projections in the monkey and human fetal cerebrum revealed by transient cholinesterase staining. J Neurosci. 1984;4(1):25-42.
32. Joseph R. Fetal brain behavior and cognitive development. Dev Rev. 2000;20(1):81-98.
33. Prechtl HF, Einspieler C. Is neurological assessment of the fetus possible? Eur J Obstet Gynecol Reprod Biol. 1997;75(1):81-4.
34. Hadders-Algra M, Klip-Van den Nieuwendijk A, Martijn A, et al. Assessment of general movements: towards a better understanding of a sensitive method to evaluate brain function in young infants. Dev Med Child Neurol. 1997;39(2):88-98.
35. Salihagić-Kadić A, Medić M, Kurjak A. Neurophysiology of fetal behavior. Ultrasound Rev Obstet Gynecol. 2004;4(1):2-11.
36. Kurjak A, Carrera JM, Andonotopo W, et al. Behavioral perinatology assessed by four-dimensional sonography. Perinatal Med. 2003;42:582-8.
37. Araki M, Nishitani S, Ushimaru K, et al. Fetal response to induced maternal emotions. J Physiol Sci. 2010;60(3):213-20.
38. Marybeth Grant-Beuttler, Glynn LM, Salisbury AL, et al. Development of fetal movement between 26 and 36-weeks' gestation in response to vibro-acoustic stimulation. Front Psychol, 2011;2:350.
39. DeBoer T, Wewerka S, Bauer PJ, et al. Explicit memory performance in infants of diabetic mothers at 1 year of age. Dev Med Child Neurol. 2005;47(8):525-31.
40. Cioni G, Prechtl HF, Ferrari F, et al. Which better predicts later outcome in full-term infants: quality of general movements or neurological examination? Early Hum Dev. 1997;50(1):71-85.
41. Widness JA, Susa JB, Garcia JF, et al. Increased erythropoiesis and elevated erythropoietin in infants born to diabetic mothers and in hyperinsulinemic rhesus fetuses. J Clin Invest. 1981;67(3):637-42.
42. Petry CD, Eaton MA, Wobken JD, et al. Iron deficiency of liver, heart, and brain in newborn infants of diabetic mothers. J Pediatr. 1992;121(1):109-14.
43. Barks JD, Sun R, Malinak C, et al. gp120, an HIV-1 protein, increases susceptibility to hypoglycemic and ischemic brain injury in perinatal rats. Exp Neurol. 1995;132(1):123-33.
44. Mills JL. Malformations in infants of diabetic mothers. Birth Defects Res A Clin Mol Teratol. 2010;88(10):769-78.

45. de Deungria M, Rao R, Wobken JD, et al. Perinatal iron deficiency decreases cytochrome c oxidase (CytOx) activity in selected regions of neonatal rat brain. Pediatr Res. 2000;48(2):169-76.

46. Churchill JA, Berendes HW, Nemore J. Neuropsychological deficits in children of diabetic mothers. A report from the Collaborative Study of Cerebral Palsy. Am J Obstet Gynecol. 1969;105(2):257-68.

47. Stehbens JA, Baker GL, Kitchell M. Outcome at ages 1, 3, and 5 years of children born to diabetic women. Am J Obstet Gynecol. 1977;127(4):408-13.

48. Felig P, Marliss E, Ohman JL, et al. Plasma amino acid levels in diabetic ketoacidosis. Diabetes. 1970;19(10):727-8.

49. Jovanovic L, Peterson CM, Saxena BB, et al. Feasibility of maintaining normal glucose profiles in insulin-dependent pregnant diabetic women. Am J Med. 1980;68(1):105-12.

50. Morokuma S, Fukushima K, Yumoto Y, et al. Simplified ultrasound screening for fetal brain function based on behavioral pattern. Early Hum Dev. 2007;83(3):177-81.

51. Horimoto N, Koyanagi T, Maeda H, et al. Can brain impairment be detected by in utero behavioral patterns? Arch Dis Child. 1993;69(1 Spec No):3-8.

52. Kurjak A, Andonotopo W, Hafner T, et al. Normal standards for fetal neurobehavioral developments: longitudinal quantification by four-dimensional sonography. J Perinat Med. 2006;34(1):56-65.

53. Nijhuis JG, Prechtl HF, Martin CB, et al. Are there behavioral states in the human fetus? Early Hum Dev. 1982;6(2):177-95.

54. Stanojevic M, Antsaklis P, Kadic AS, et al. Is Kurjak antenatal neurodevelopmental test ready for routine clinical application? Bucharest Consensus Statement. DSJUOG. 2015;9(3):260-5.

55. Rosier-van Dunné FM, van Wezel-Meijler G, Bakker MP, et al. Fetal general movements and brain sonography in a population at risk for preterm birth. Early Hum Dev. 2010;86(2):107-11.

56. Kurjak A, Stanojevic M, Andonotopo W, et al. Fetal behavior assessed in all three trimesters of normal pregnancy by four-dimensional ultrasonography. Croat Med J. 2005;46(5):772-80.

57. Stanojevic M, Talic A, Miskovic B, et al. An attempt to standardize Kurjak's antenatal neurodevelopmental test: Osaka Consensus Statement. DSJUOG. 2011;5(4):317-29.

58. Low JA, Galbraith RS, Muir DW, et al. Factors associated with motor and cognitive deficits in children after intrapartum fetal hypoxia. Am J Obstet Gynecol. 1984;148(5):533-9.

59. Kurjak A, Miskovic B, Stanojevic M, et al. New scoring system for fetal neurobehavior assessed by three- and four-dimensional sonography. J Perinat Med. 2008;36(1):73-81.

60. Nelson C, Silverstein FS. Acute disruption of cytochrome oxidase activity in brain in a perinatal rat stroke model. Pediatr Res. 1994;36(1 Pt 1):12-9.

61. Visser GH, Mulder EJ, Tessa Ververs FF. Fetal behavioral teratology. J Matern Fetal Neonatal Med. 2010;23 Suppl 3:14-6.

62. Visser GH, Bekedam DJ, Mulder EJ, et al. Delayed emergence of fetal behavior in type-1 diabetic women. Early Hum Dev. 1985;12(2):167-72.

63. Aladjem S, Feria A, Rest J, et al. Effect of maternal glucose load on fetal activity. Am J Obstet Gynecol. 1979;134(3):276-80.

64. Eller DP, Stramm SL, Newman RB. The effect of maternal intravenous glucose administration on fetal activity. Am J Obstet Gynecol. 1992;167(4 Pt 1):1071-4.

65. Gelman SR, Spellacy WN, Wood S, et al. Fetal movements and ultrasound: effect of maternal intravenous glucose administration. Am J Obstet Gynecol. 1980;137(4):459-61.

66. Goodman JD. The effect of intravenous glucose on human fetal breathing measured by Doppler ultrasound. Br J Obstet Gynecol. 1980;87(12):1080-3.

67. Miller FC, Skiba H, Klapholz H. The effect of maternal blood sugar levels on fetal activity. Obstet Gynecol. 1978;52(6):662-5.

68. Richardson B, Briggs ML, Toomey C, et al. The effect of maternal glucose administration on the specificity of the nonstress test. Am J Obstet Gynecol. 1983;145(2):141-6.

69. Allen CL, Kisilevsky BS. Fetal behavior in diabetic and nondiabetic pregnant women: An exploratory study. Dev Psychobiol. 1999;35(1):69-80.

70. Edelberg SC, Dierker L, Kalhan S, et al. Decreased fetal movements with sustained maternal hyperglycemia using the glucose clamp technique. Am J Obstet Gynecol. 1987;156(5):1101-5.
71. Holden KP, Jovanovic L, Druzin ML, et al. Increased fetal activity with low maternal blood glucose levels in pregnancies complicated by diabetes. Am J Perinatol. 1984;1(2):161-4.
72. Bocking AD. Observations of biophysical activities in the normal fetus. Clin Perinatol. 1989;16(3):583-94.
73. Bocking A, Adamson L, Carmichael L, et al. Effect of intravenous glucose injection on human maternal and fetal heart rate at term. Am J Obstet Gynecol. 1984;148(4):414-20.
74. Bocking A, Adamson L, Cousin A, et al. Effects of intravenous glucose injections on human fetal breathing movements and gross fetal body movements at 38 to 40 weeks' gestational age. Am J Obstet Gynecol. 1982;142(6 Pt 1):606-11.
75. Reece EA, Hagay Z, Roberts AB, et al. Fetal Doppler and behavioral responses during hypoglycemia induced with the insulin clamp technique in pregnant diabetic women. Am J Obstet Gynecol. 1995;172(1 Pt 1):151-5.
76. Patrick J, Campbell K, Carmichael L, et al. Patterns of gross fetal body movements over 24-hour observation intervals during the last 10 weeks of pregnancy. Am J Obstet Gynecol. 1982;142(4): 363-71.
77. Ornoy A, Ratzon N, Greenbaum C, et al. Neurobehavior of school age children born to diabetic mothers. Arch Dis Child Fetal Neonatal Ed. 1998;79(2):F94-9.
78. Wolf A. Developmental Evaluation on Early School Age Children Born to Gestational Diabetic Mothers. Israel: Hebrew University; 1997.
79. Mulder EJ, Leiblum DM, Visser GH. Fetal breathing movements in late diabetic pregnancy: relationship to fetal heart rate patterns and Braxton Hicks' contractions. Early Hum Dev. 1995;43(3): 225-32.
80. Schulte FJ, Michaelis R, Nolte R, et al. Brain and behavioral maturation in newborn infants of diabetic mothers. I. Nerve conduction and EEG patterns. Neuropadiatrie. 1969;1(1):24-35.
81. Robertson SS, Dierker LJ. Fetal cyclic motor activity in diabetic pregnancies: sensitivity to maternal blood glucose. Dev Psychobiol. 2003;42(1):9-16.
82. Devoe LD, Youssef AA, Castillo RA, et al. Fetal biophysical activities in third-trimester pregnancies complicated by diabetes mellitus. Am J Obstet Gynecol. 1994;171(2):298-303.
83. Dierker LJ, Pillay S, Sorokin Y, et al. The change in fetal activity periods in diabetic and nondiabetic pregnancies. Am J Obstet Gynecol. 1982;143(2):181-5.
84. Doherty NN, Hepper PG. Habituation in fetuses of diabetic mothers. Early Hum Dev. 2000;59(2): 85-93.
85. Kainer F, Prechtl HF, Engele H, et al. Assessment of the quality of general movements in fetuses and infants of women with type-1 diabetes mellitus. Early Hum Dev. 1997;50(1):13-25.
86. Mulder EJ, O'Brien MJ, Lems YL, et al. Body and breathing movements in near-term fetuses and newborn infants of type-1 diabetic women. Early Hum Dev. 1990;24(2):131-52.
87. Mulder EJ, Visser GH. Growth and motor development in fetuses of women with type-1 diabetes. I. Early growth patterns. Early Hum Dev. 1991;25(2):91-106.
88. Mulder EJ, Visser GH. Growth and motor development in fetuses of women with type-1 diabetes. II. Emergence of specific movement patterns. Early Hum Dev. 1991;25(2):107-15.
89. Mulder EJ, Visser GH. Impact of early growth delay on subsequent fetal growth and functional development: a study on diabetic pregnancy. Early Hum Dev. 1992;31(2):91-5.
90. Mulder EJ, Visser GH, Bekedam DJ, et al. Emergence of behavioral states in fetuses of type-1 diabetic women. Early Hum Dev. 1987;15(4):231-51.
91. Mulder EJ, Visser GH, Morssink LP, et al. Growth and motor development in fetuses of women with type-1 diabetes. III. First trimester quantity of fetal movement patterns. Early Hum Dev. 1991;25(2):117-33.
92. Aberg A, Westbom L, Källén B. Congenital malformations among infants whose mothers had gestational diabetes or preexisting diabetes. Early Hum Dev. 2001;61(2):85-95.

93. Deregnier RA, Nelson CA, Thomas KM, et al. Neurophysiologic evaluation of auditory recognition memory in healthy newborn infants and infants of diabetic mothers. J Pediatr. 2000;137(6):777-84.
94. Nelson CA, Wewerka S, Thomas KM, et al. Neurocognitive sequelae of infants of diabetic mothers. Behav Neurosci. 2000;114(5):950-6.
95. Reece EA, Homko CJ. Infant of the diabetic mother. Semin Perinatol. 1994;18:459-69.
96. Reece EA, Homko CJ. Why do diabetic women deliver malformed infants? Clin Obstet Gynecol. 2000;43(1):32-45.
97. Rizzo T, Metzger BE, Burns WJ, et al. Correlations between antepartum maternal metabolism and intelligence of offspring. N Engl J Med. 1991;325(13):911-6.
98. Rizzo TA, Metzger BE, Dooley SL, et al. Early malnutrition and child neurobehavioral development: insights from the study of children of diabetic mothers. Child Dev. 1997;68(1):26-38.
99. Schwartz R, Teramo KA. Effects of diabetic pregnancy on the fetus and newborn. Semin Perinatol. 2000;24(2):120-35.
100. Vääräsmäki MS, Hartikainen A, Anttila M, et al. Factors predicting peri- and neonatal outcome in diabetic pregnancy. Early Hum Dev. 2000;59(1):61-70.
101. Robertson SS, Dierker LJ. Fetal cyclic motor activity in diabetic pregnancies: sensitivity to maternal blood glucose. Dev Psychobiol. 2003;42(1):9-16.
102. Accardo PJ, Blondis TA, Whitman BY. Disorders of attention and activity level in a referral population. Pediatrics. 1990;85(3 Pt 2):426-31.
103. Ornoy A, Uriel L, Tennenbaum A. Inattention, hyperactivity and speech delay at 2-4 years of age as a predictor for ADD-ADHD syndrome. Isr J Psychiatry Relat Sci. 1993;30(3):155-63.
104. Smyth TR. Impaired motor skill (clumsiness) in otherwise normal children: a review. Child Care Health Dev. 1992;18(5):283-300.
105. Petersen MB, Pedersen SA, Greisen G, et al. Early growth delay in diabetic pregnancy: relation to psychomotor development at age 4. Br Med J (Clin Res Ed). 1988;296(6622):598-600.
106. Sells CJ, Robinson NM, Brown Z, et al. Long-term developmental follow-up of infants of diabetic mothers. J Pediatr. 1994;125(1):S9-17.
107. Vladareanu R, Lebit D, Constantinescu S. Ultrasound assessment of fetal neurobehaviour in high-risk pregnancies. DSJUOG. 2012;6(2):132-47.
108. Talic A, Kurjak A, Ahmed B, et al. The potential of 4D sonography in the assessment of fetal behavior in high-risk pregnancies. J Matern Fetal Neonatal Med. 2011;24(7):948-54.
109. Bekedam DJ, Visser GH, de Vries JJ, et al. Motor behaviour in the growth retarded fetus. Early Hum Dev. 1985;12(2):155-65.
110. Cioni G, Prechtl HF. Preterm and early postterm motor behaviour in low-risk premature infants. Early Hum Dev. 1990;23(3):159-91.
111. Seme-Ciglenecki P. Predictive value of assessment of general movements for neurological development of high-risk preterm infants: comparative study. Croat Med J. 2003;44(6):721-7.
112. Abo-Yaqoub S, Kurjak A, Mohammed AB, et al. The role of 4-D ultrasonography in prenatal assessment of fetal neurobehaviour and prediction of neurological outcome. J Matern Fetal Neonatal Med. 2012;25(3):231-6.
113. Athanasiadis AP, Mikos T, Tambakoudis GP, et al. Neurodevelopmental fetal assessment using KANET scoring system in low and high-risk pregnancies. J Matern Fetal Neonatal Med. 2013;26(4):363-8.

# Chapter 5

# Overview of the Role of Ultrasound in the Management of Diabetic Pregnancy

*Sonal Panchal*

## INTRODUCTION

An association between diabetes mellitus in women and congenital malformations in their offspring has been suspected since the 19th century. Diabetes during pregnancy is associated with an increased rate of spontaneous abortions, intrauterine death, and several congenital anomalies involving different body systems of the fetus. Most studies show a generalized increase in malformations involving multiple organ systems.[1-9]

Despite better management, the incidence of congenital malformations has not decreased over the past 25 years. The incidence is directly related to the severity of the disease, and may also be related to glycosylated hemoglobin (HbA1c) blood concentrations.[10-13]

This is why the prognosis for these patients significantly improved after the invention of insulin for diabetes control. Over the past 10–15 years, there seems to have been a significant reduction in the prevalence of congenital anomalies among the children of diabetic mothers. Close monitoring of these pregnancies by ultrasound has significantly improved the prognosis for these fetuses. This is directly related to the improvement in glycemic control during early pregnancy. The rate of congenital anomalies has significantly reduced in well-treated diabetic pregnant women.[4,7]

- Results of a study from Netherlands showed 84% (n = 271) of the pregnancies were planned. Glycemic control early in pregnancy was good in most women [HbA1c 7.0% in 75% (n = 212) of the population], and folic acid supplementation was adequate in 70% (n = 226). 314 pregnancies that went beyond 24 weeks' gestation resulted in 324 infants. The rates of preeclampsia (40; 12.7%), preterm delivery (101; 32.2%), cesarean section (139; 44.3%), maternal mortality (2; 0.6%), congenital malformations (29; 8.8%), perinatal mortality (9; 2.8%), and macrosomia (146; 45.1%) were considerably higher than in the general population. Neonatal morbidity (one or more complications) was extremely high (260; 80.2%). The incidence of major congenital malformations was significantly lower in planned pregnancies than in unplanned pregnancies [4.2% (n = 11) vs 12.2% (n = 6); relative risk 0.34, 95% confidence interval (CI) 0.13–0.88].

Complications probably are not present in women whose diabetes can be controlled by diet or oral hypoglycemic agents. The cause though is not surely known.[1]

## INCIDENCE

Moltsed-Pedersen et al. examined 853 consecutive infants of diabetic mothers and compared them to 1,212 infants of nondiabetic mothers and showed that frequency of major (including fatal) and total malformations was three times higher in the diabetic group. Fatal malformations and malformations involving several organ systems were approximately six times more frequent in the diabetics.[15] Kucera et al. found that abnormalities of the skeleton, kidneys, heart, gastrointestinal system, and genitalia all occurred significantly more frequently in infants of diabetic mothers.[16]

It has been shown in a study of 392 women with gestational diabetes by Collaborative Perinatal Project that fetal malformation rates were 15.3% for whites and 13.7% for blacks. The corresponding rates for nondiabetics were 14.6 and 17.0%, respectively. The differences were not significant.[17]

Congenital anomalies are more common (2.5–12%) in fetuses of diabetic women as compared to euglycemic women and the cardiac anomalies have the highest incidence.[18,19] Studies in women with pre-existing diabetes (type 1 or type 2) and a pre-pregnancy body mass index (BMI) equal to 28 kg/m$^2$ have shown a three-fold increase (adjusted rates) in the risk of congenital abnormalities (excluding second trimester terminations of pregnancy).[20]

The risk of major malformations is markedly increased in infants of diabetic mothers, ranging from 4% to 10%, which is two- to three-fold higher than in the general population, with even higher absolute and relative risks for particular malformations, such as neural tube defects (1% risk).[21]

Population-based prospective cohort studies that include second trimester terminations of pregnancy have demonstrated a 1.7- to 3-fold increase in risk of congenital abnormalities in women with type 1 diabetes. Poorer the glucose control periconceptionally or in early pregnancy, the greater the risk for congenital anomalies.[22-27]

Though maternal insulin-dependent diabetes has long been associated with congenital malformations, it is not as common with gestational diabetes. Gestational diabetes is a group of glucose intolerant conditions that has its onset or is first recognized during pregnancy and complicates 2–4% of all pregnancies.[28-31] Anomalies for gestational diabetes are 1.2 times higher than in the total population (95% CI 1.1–1.3).[32] A 3.4-fold increase in anomalies for women with gestational diabetes with fasting hyperglycemia.[33] In women with gestational diabetes, increasing hyperglycemia at diagnosis was associated with an increasing risk of anomalies. Therefore, women at high risk for gestational diabetes may benefit from early glucose screening.[34]

Though according to some studies, congenital malformations have now replaced respiratory distress syndrome as the leading cause of death in some diabetes centers.[35,36]

## CAUSATIVE MECHANISM

Congenital malformations in the fetuses are even more common in fetuses of those females who were already on insulin at the time of conception. It is thought that maternal diabetes, via its effects on maternal metabolism, is responsible for the increase of malformations in the offspring.[37]

Diabetes is responsible for a loss of normal homeostasis not only of carbohydrate but of fat and protein metabolism as well. Vascular complications may lead to additional metabolic changes such as hypoxia or impaired renal clearance of toxins. In short, there are multiple factors in the disordered milieu of the pregnant diabetic which could be teratogenic. The most important human data on hyperglycemia and malformations come from recent reports of HbA1c levels in early pregnancy. Since HbA1c represents an integrated measure of blood glucose over the preceding weeks, elevation of HbA1c in the second or third month of pregnancy is a fair indicator of hyperglycemia during organogenesis.[1]

The malformation rate in infants whose mothers' HbA1c had been 8.5 or less was 3.4%; the malformation rate in infants whose mothers' HbA1c had been over 8.5 was remarkable 22.4%.[5]

## BIOCHEMICAL PARAMETERS

First trimester marker, pregnancy-associated plasma protein-A (PAPP-A) is reduced in insulin-dependent diabetes mellitus (IDDM) mothers.[38]

In pre-existing or gestational diabetes, free beta-human chorionic gonadotropin (β-hCG) and PAPP-A are reduced by 20% and 25%, respectively.[39] Among the second trimester markers, in IDDM mothers, alpha-fetoprotein (AFP) has inverse relationship with glycosylated heamoglobin.[40] It is these markers that may be representative of the congenital fetal anomalies seen in the diabetic mothers.

## MALFORMATIONS

Diabetic embryopathy, a spectrum of congenital malformations or disruptions considered to be caused by maternal diabetes mellitus, is a diagnosis of exclusion.[41] Small but statistically significant increase in holoprosencephaly (HPE), costovertebral, and genitourinary (GU) tract anomalies in offspring of women with gestational diabetes compared with women without diabetes.[33]

In the offspring of women with pre-existing diabetes, the incidence of cardiovascular abnormalities ranges from 2 to 34 per 1,000 births, central nervous system abnormalities from 1 to 5 per 1,000 births, musculoskeletal abnormalities from 2 to 20 per 1,000 births, GU abnormalities from 2 to 32 per 1,000 births, and gastrointestinal abnormalities from 1 to 5 per 1,000 births.[32,42,43]

List of fetal conditions associated with maternal diabetes:[32,42,44]

- *Cardiac*: congenital cardiac anomalies
  - Ventricular septal defect (VSD)
  - Conotruncal anomalies
    - Transposition of the great arteries (TGA)
    - Truncus arteriosus
  - Hyperplastic cardiomyopathy and aortic stenosis
  - Fetal congestive cardiac failure (without any structural cardiac anomaly)
  - Situs inversus
  - Single ventricle
  - Hypoplastic left ventricle
- Pulmonary
  - Surfactant deficiency
  - Transient tachypnea of the newborn (TTN)
- Central nervous system
  - Neural tube defects: anencephaly, meningomyelocele, etc.

- Spina bifida, encephaloceles, etc.
- Holoprosencephaly
- Caudal regression syndrome
- Sirenomelia
■ Gastrointestinal
  - Situs anomalies
  - Meconium plug syndrome
  - Rectal atresia
  - Small left colon
■ Renal
  - Renal agenesis
  - Fetal hydronephrosis
  - Ureteric duplication
  - Multicystic dysplasia
■ Skeletal
  - Polydactyly
  - Syndactyly
  - Focal femoral hypoplasia
■ Others
  - Polyhydramnios
  - Large for dates fetus
  - Fetal macrosomia
  - *Intrauterine growth restriction (IUGR)*: When the maternal diabetes is severe there can be a paradoxical IUGR as opposed to fetal macrosomia
  - Single umbilical artery
  - Dysplastic external ears and oculo-auriculo-vertebral spectrum.[45]

## Cardiac Anomalies

With congenital heart disease occurring in up to 5% of fetuses of diabetic mothers, and with 90% of the cardiac lesions identifiable prenatally, it has been suggested that detailed fetal echocardiography is offered to all diabetic women during pregnancy.[46-50]

The most frequent cardiac anomalies in infants of diabetic mothers (IDMs) include VSD, transposition of great arteries, and aortic stenosis. Defects involving the great arteries, including truncus arteriosus and double outlet right ventricle, are also more prevalent in IDMs.[51,52]

### Ventricular Septal Defect

Best seen on four-chamber heart if muscular VSD is present. Lateral four-chamber view is the best to diagnose these defects and shows drop out in septal shadow. But small defects are difficult to diagnose without color Doppler. On apical and basal four-chamber view, the part of the septum close to the crux is often not seen (Fig. 5.1). This must not be misinterpreted as septal defect. It is a defect only if the end of the septal line shows a thickened end otherwise it is an artifact (Fig. 5.2).

Color Doppler may be used to define these defects. Even on color Doppler no turbulence will be seen as there is no pressure gradient between both chambers. The flow may be left-to-right or right-to-left (Fig. 5.3).

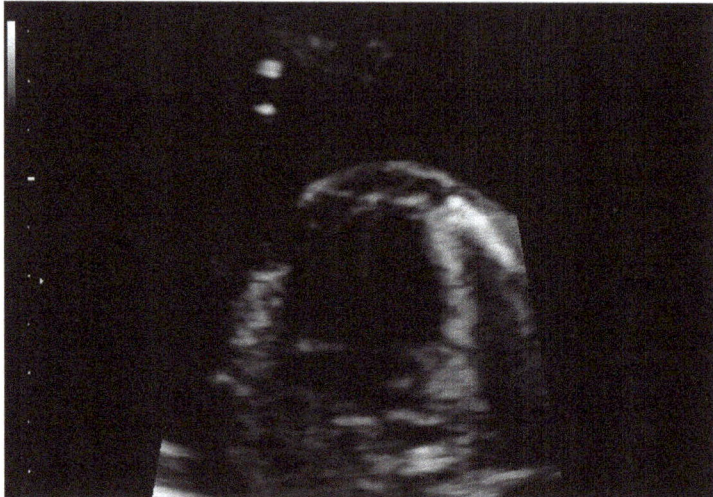

**Fig. 5.1:** Apical four-chamber view of the heart showing a small gap in the ventricular septal shadow, just apical to the atrioventricular (AV) valves. The ventricular septal line tapers and disappears, just apical to AV valves.

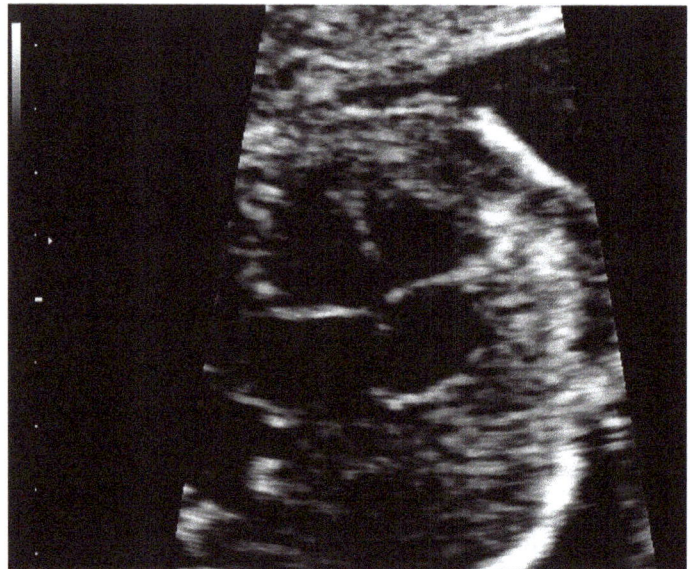

**Fig. 5.2:** Apical four-chamber view of the heart showing a small gap in the ventricular septal shadow, just apical to the atrioventricular (AV) valves. The ventricular septal line shows a sharp cutoff just apical to AV valves— ventricular septal defect (VSD).

## Conotruncal Anomalies

For diagnosis of conotruncal anomalies, detailed study of outflow tracts is essential. At a level above the four-chamber view of the heart the left ventricular outflow tract is seen (Fig. 5.4).

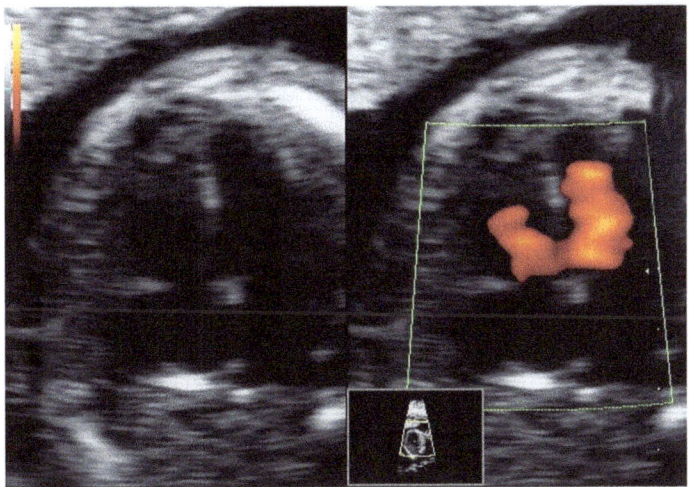

**Fig. 5.3:** B-mode and power Doppler images of the ventricular septal defect—B-mode showing a sharp cutoff of the ventricular septal shadow and power Doppler shows flow across this defect.

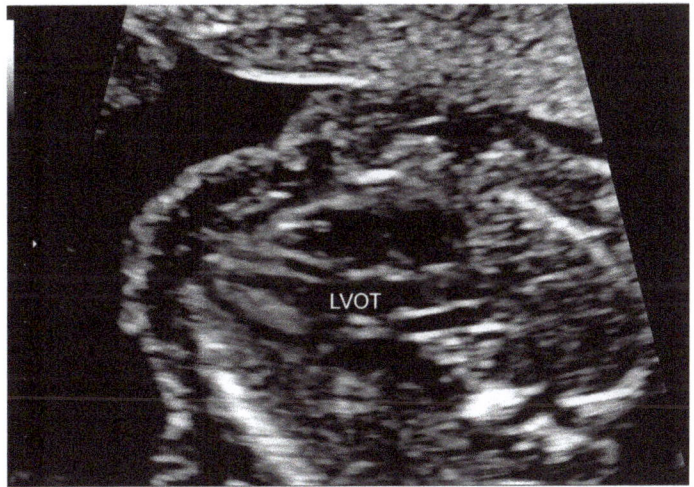

**Fig. 5.4:** B-mode image of the left ventricular outflow tract (LVOT).

It runs oblique towards right from the left ventricle and then curves to left to join the pulmonary trunk at ductus arteriosus. As it curves in the aortic arch it gives three-neck branches (Fig. 5.5). At the origin its medial wall is continuous with the interventricular septum—this is the membranous part of the septum and its lateral wall appears in continuity with the cusp of the mitral valve.

The right ventricular outflow tract is seen superior to the left ventricular outflow tract, arising from the right ventricle, taking a straight course and dividing into two main branches (Fig. 5.6). Both the outflow tracts cross over each other (Fig. 5.7).

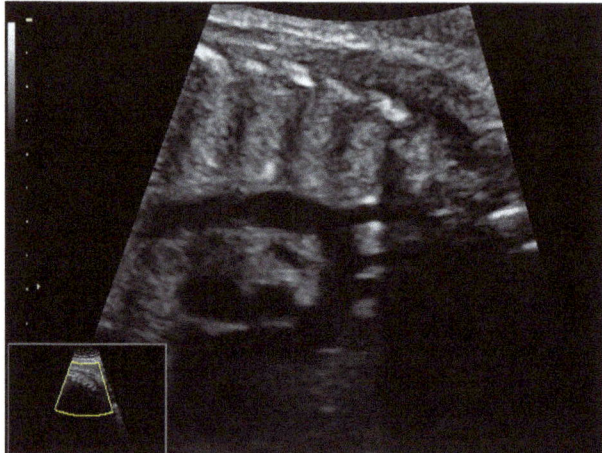

**Fig. 5.5:** B-mode image of the aortic arch in sagittal section.

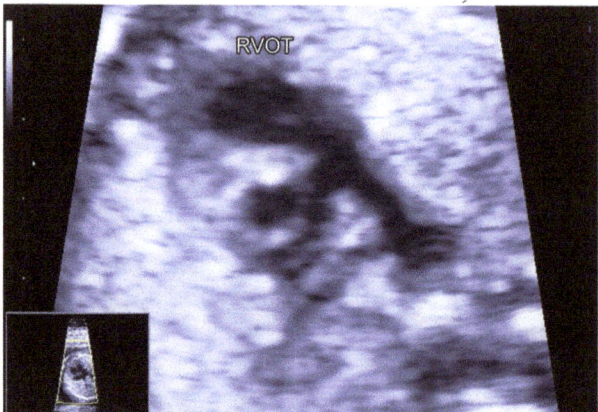

**Fig. 5.6:** B-mode image of the right ventricular outflow tract (RVOT) showing bifurcation.

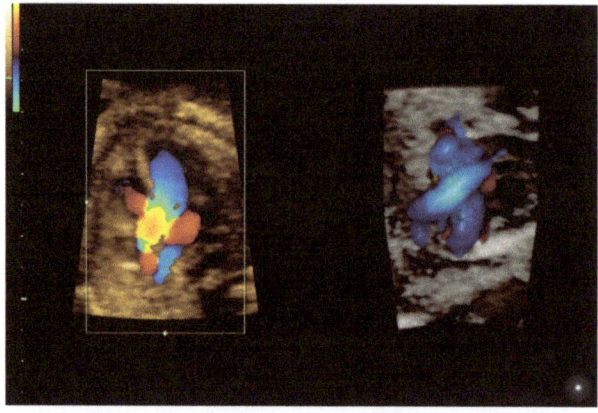

**Fig. 5.7:** Color Doppler showing crossing over of right and left outflow tracts.

It is important to confirm the ventriculoarterial concordance and cross over to exclude conotruncal anomalies.

*Transposition of great vessels*: In this abnormality, aorta arises from right ventricle and lies anteriorly and to left of pulmonary trunk and pulmonary trunk arises from left ventricle. This means two great arteries arise side-by-side at the base of the heart instead of crossing over of great vessels (Fig. 5.8).

On ultrasound normal four-chamber view is seen. Outflow tracts show parallel great vessels at the roots. There is no crossing over of vessels. Vessel arising out of left ventricle (LV) takes posterior course and bifurcates so is pulmonary artery. Vessel arising out of right ventricle (RV) takes long upward course and curves. This is aorta (Fig. 5.9). If associated with VSD and overriding, the diagnosis is difficult.

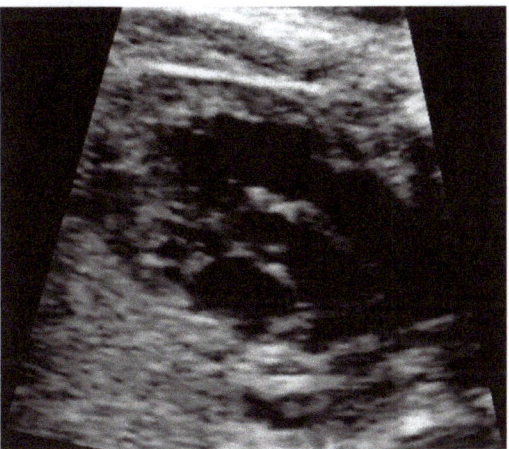

**Fig. 5.8:** B-mode image showing two outflow tracts parallel to each other (this is not normal and is unlike the normal crossover of outflow tracts).

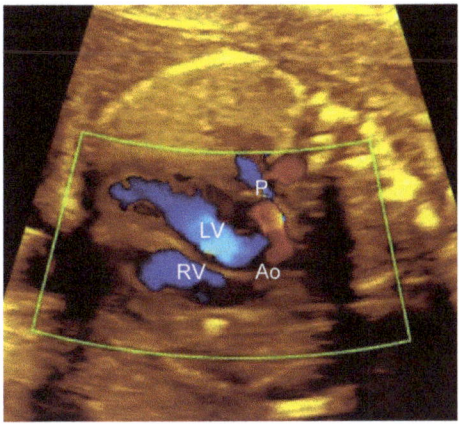

**Fig. 5.9:** Color Doppler showing two parallel outflow tracts. The outflow tract originating from right ventricle (RV) curves and the one from the left ventricle (LV) bifurcates, indicating transposition of great vessels. (Ao: Aorta; PA: Pulmonary artery).

*Truncus arteriosus*: Both the arteries arise as a single trunk from the ventricles. It is usually associated with a large VSD with the trunk overriding the septum (Fig. 5.10). Truncus may give out the main pulmonary trunk that divides into two pulmonary arteries or the pulmonary arteries may arise individually from the truncus. When these arise individually, these may arise from two sides of truncus or may arise from the truncus, anteriorly and posteriorly.

On ultrasound increased cardiac axis is seen on otherwise normal four-chamber view. Malaligned large VSD is seen in outlet part of ventricular septum (Fig. 5.11). Truncal root is seen arising from RV or overriding the septum. Abnormal truncal valve may or may not be present. The origin of pulmonary artery (PA) must be confirmed to exclude pulmonary stenosis.

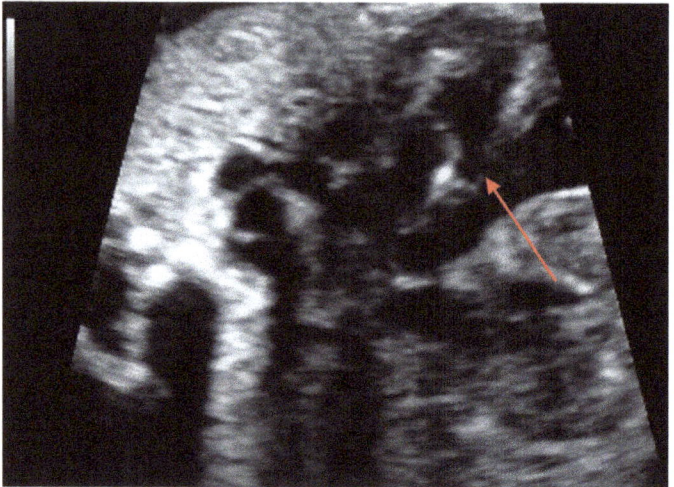

**Fig. 5.10:** B-mode image of the heart showing single outflow tract arising over the ventricular septum with a large ventricular septal defect (VSD) as shown by the arrow.

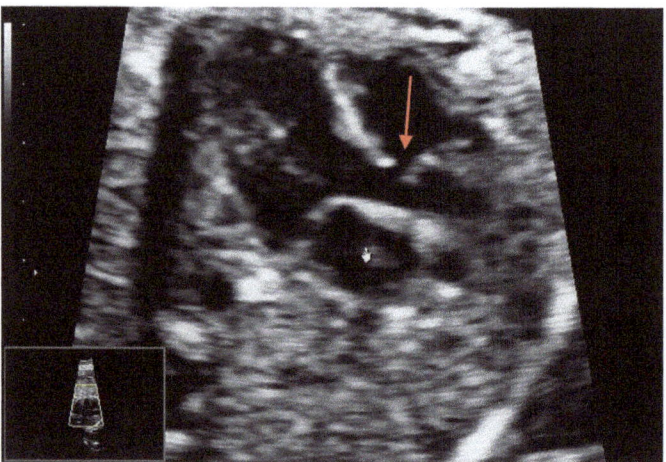

**Fig. 5.11:** B-mode image of the left ventricular outflow tract with a malaligned ventricular septal defect (VSD) as shown by the arrow.

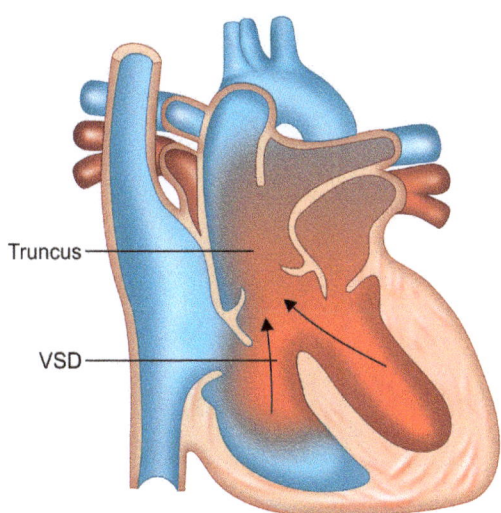

**Fig. 5.12:** Diagrammatic presentation of the truncus arteriosus—a single outflow tract—showing the origin of the pulmonary trunk that divides into two. (VSD: Ventricular septal defect)

On color Doppler VSD is seen with origin of truncus overriding the septum. Origin of pulmonary artery from the main trunk must be confirmed (Fig. 5.12). This is important because even with an overriding of aorta and large aortic root there may be compression and stenosis of the pulmonary artery. This condition appears very similar on ultrasound to truncus arteriosus with the only difference that the pulmonary trunk is not seen arising from the aorta or the main trunk. If dysplastic valve is present, it shows holodiastolic regurgitation on pulse Doppler.

## Septal Hypertrophy

In fetuses of diabetic mothers, along with other congenital heart defects, hypertrophic septal cardiomyopathy is especially common.[53,54]

It is believed that maternal hyperglycemia leads to fetal hyperinsulinemia that has an anabolic effect and leads to macrosomia, but more often to septal hypertrophy. It may be found in up to 30% of the fetuses of diabetic mothers.[55]

Hypertrophic cardiomyopathy (HC) is seen in infants of diabetic mothers, and can also be diagnosed antenatally (Fig. 5.13). Cardiomyopathy involves the left ventricle more commonly but right ventricle may also be involved sometimes. The ventricular wall is also thickened but still the systolic function is good and the circulation may also be hyperdynamic at times. There is asymmetrically increased thickness of the septum, leading to apposition of the anterior leaflet of the mitral valve to the interventricular septum during systole, leading to left ventricular outflow tract (LVOT) obstruction and in turn decreased cardiac output.[56] There may also be subvalvular aortic stenosis.[57,58] Increased ventricular wall thickness also may lead to outflow tract obstruction.[59] Fetal cardiac septum thickness should be measured in utero by sonocardiography in all diabetic pregnancies[60] (Fig. 5.14).

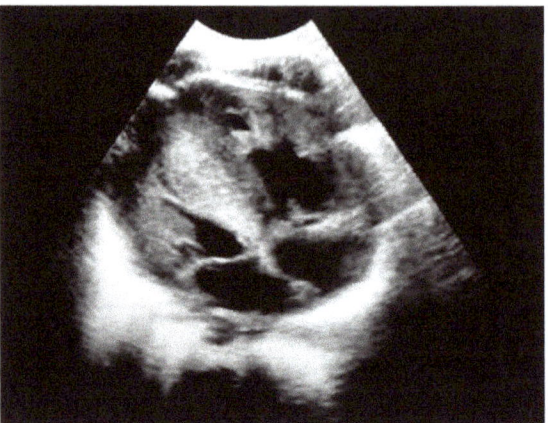

**Fig. 5.13:** B-mode image of the four-chamber heart showing thick muscular outer and lateral walls of hypertrophic cardiomyopathy.

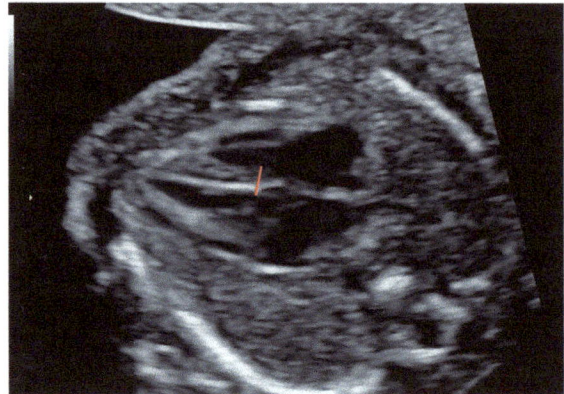

**Fig. 5.14:** B-mode ultrasound showing four-chamber heart with the red line showing the assessment of septal thickness.

The natural history of HC is that of spontaneous regression of symptoms and septal hypertrophy in 2–4 weeks, during the first 2–12 months of life.[61] But if it is progressive it has a bad prognosis.

Congestive cardiomyopathy presents as decreased cardiac contractility, reduced ejection fraction, enlarged heart and may also result into pericardial, pleural or peritoneal effusions and hydrops.

## Situs Inversus

All the viscera and the heart are on the opposite side like a mirror image (Figs. 15A and B). Heart, stomach, and aorta are on the right side and liver, gallbladder, and inferior vena cava (IVC) are on the right side of the spine. Along with this the morphological right lung is also on left side.

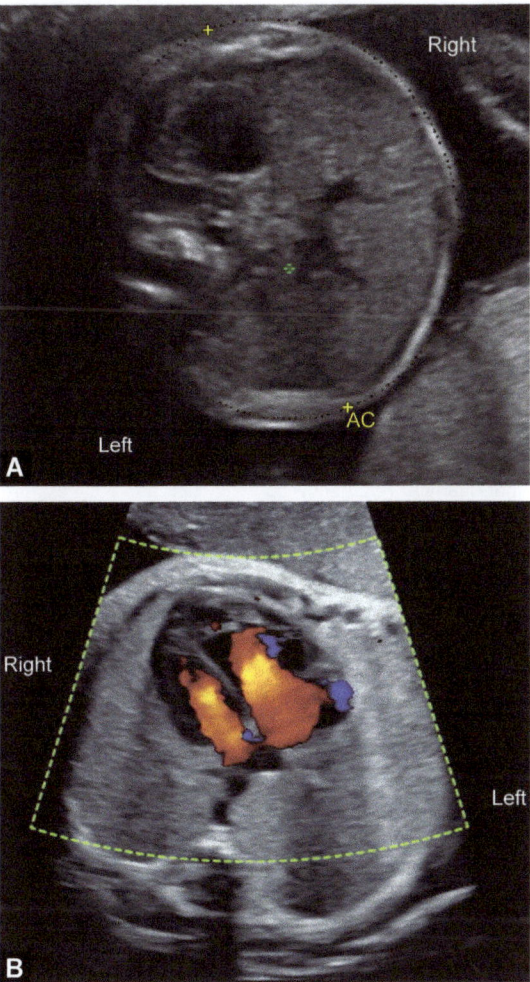

**Figs. 5.15A and B:** (A) B-mode image of the transverse section of abdomen with stomach on right side and liver on left side; (B) Color Doppler image of the four-chamber heart showing the heart placed on the right side of the thorax (AC: Abdominal circumference).

## Hypoplastic Left Heart Syndrome

Left ventricle appears small on four-chamber view with poor contractility (Fig. 5.16). Left atrium may be small or normal in size. There is no forward flow through mitral or aortic valve. Aortic size and origin site are important for postnatal prognosis. Heart may appear normal at 16–18 weeks and disease may be progressive in utero. It is important to differentiate it from single ventricle by a septal ridge in the ventricle.

## Single Ventricle Defects

Single ventricle defects especially need to be differentiated from large ventricular defects or by hypoplastic ventricle by the septal ridge or by asymmetrical ventricular wall thickness and atretic atrioventricular valve, respectively (Fig. 5.17).

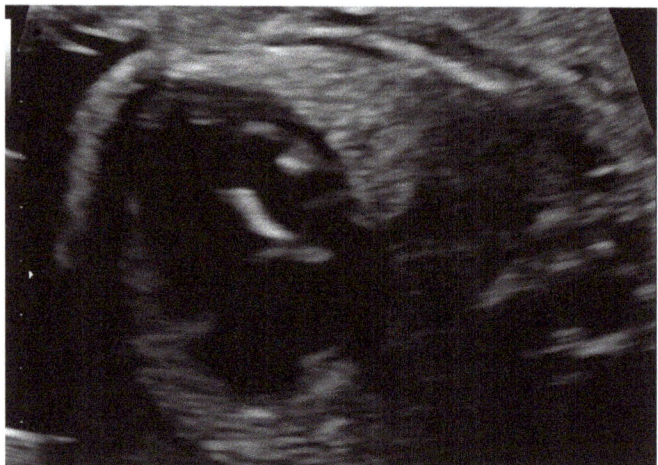

**Fig. 5.16:** B-mode image of four-chamber heart showing ventricular and atrial asymmetry with small left ventricle and small left atrium.

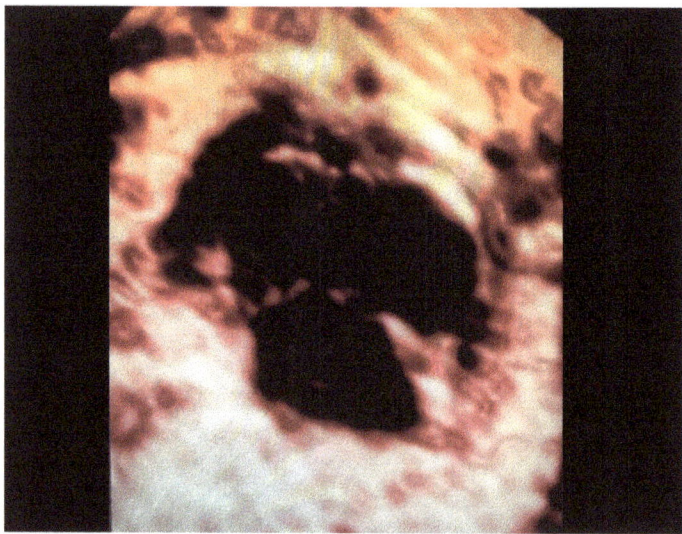

**Fig. 5.17:** B-mode ultrasound image of the heart showing single ventricular chamber with no ventricular ridge indicating a single ventricle heart.

## Central Nervous System

### *Neural Tube Defects*

These include the cranial as well as spinal defects. To list these:

- Cranial end defects
  - *Anencephaly*: It is absence of cranium and destruction of the brain matter leading to flat head and frog face due to prominent orbits (Figs. 18A and B).
  - *Iniencephaly*: Star gazing fetus (Fig. 5.19).

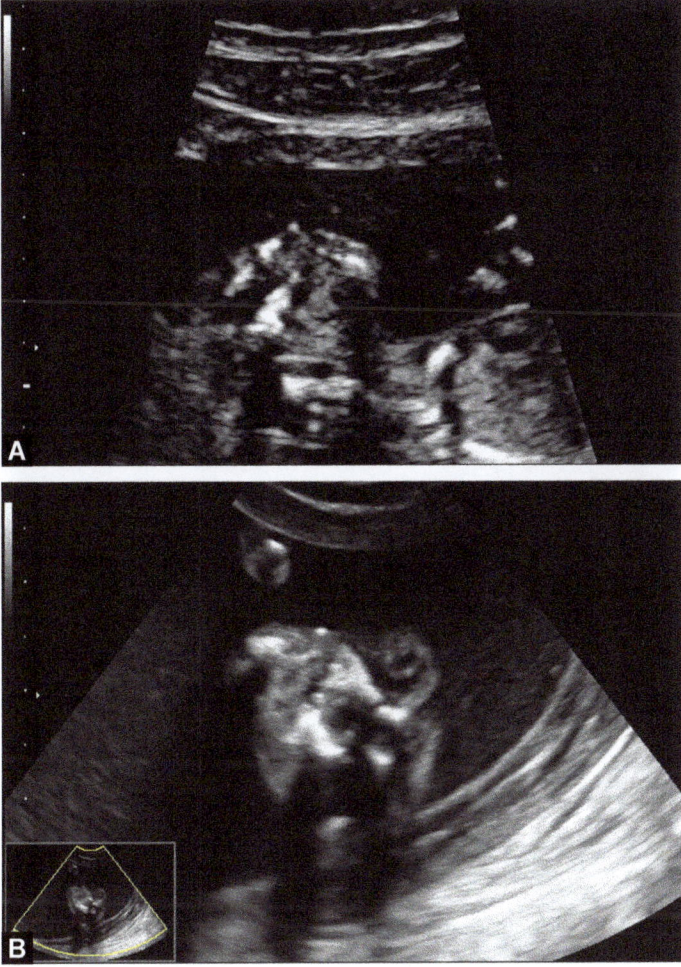

**Figs. 5.18A and B:** (A) Flat fetal head and (B) prominent orbits and absent forehead and the skull vault giving a typical frog head appearance on B-mode image.

- *Exencephaly*: Large bony defects in cranium with herniation of large part of brain (Fig. 5.20).
- *Encephalocoele*: Small defects in cranium with herniation of meninges and brain (Fig. 5.21).
- Spinal canal defects
  - Open defects with skin lesion (Fig. 5.22)
  - Closed defects without skin lesion.

Both may involve meninges (meningocele) alone or both meninges and the cord (meningomyelocele).

Spina bifida or spinal canal defects are detected by nonparallelism of the ossification centers of spinal column on coronal or sagittal section or by widening of the distance between the two ossification centers of transverse processes in individual vertebrae (Fig. 5.23). Overlying skin lesions can be best visualized on sagittal or transverse section (Fig. 5.24).

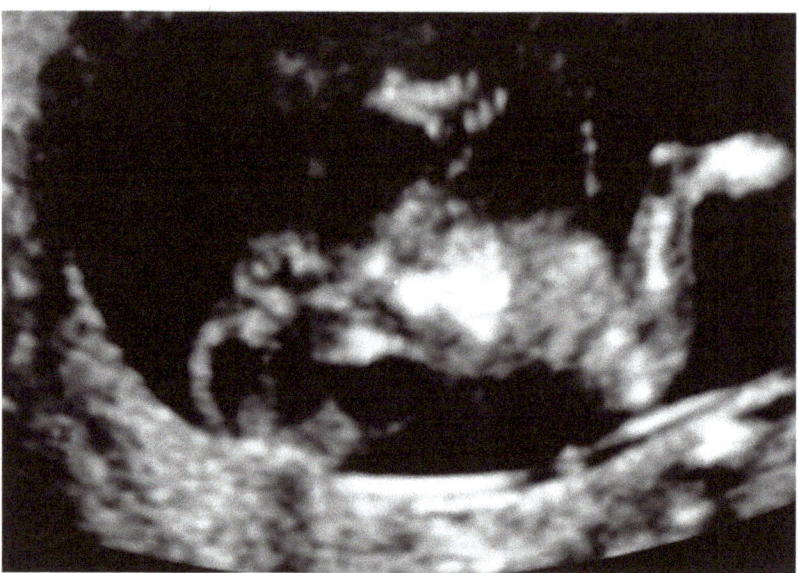

Fig. 5.19: B-mode image of the fetus with iniencephaly—a hyperextended head of the fetus.

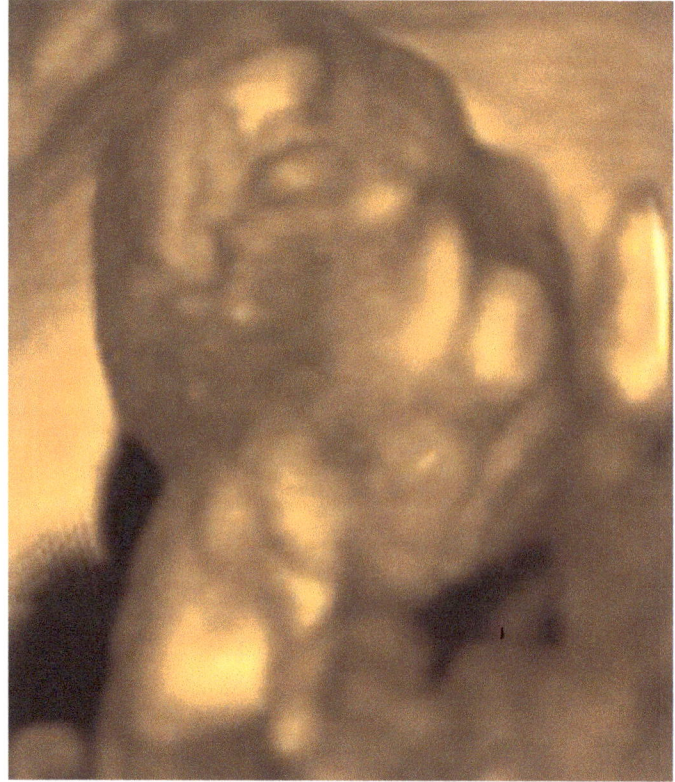

Fig. 5.20: Three-dimensional ultrasound image of the fetus with a large part of the brain herniating outside the large skull defect—exencephaly.

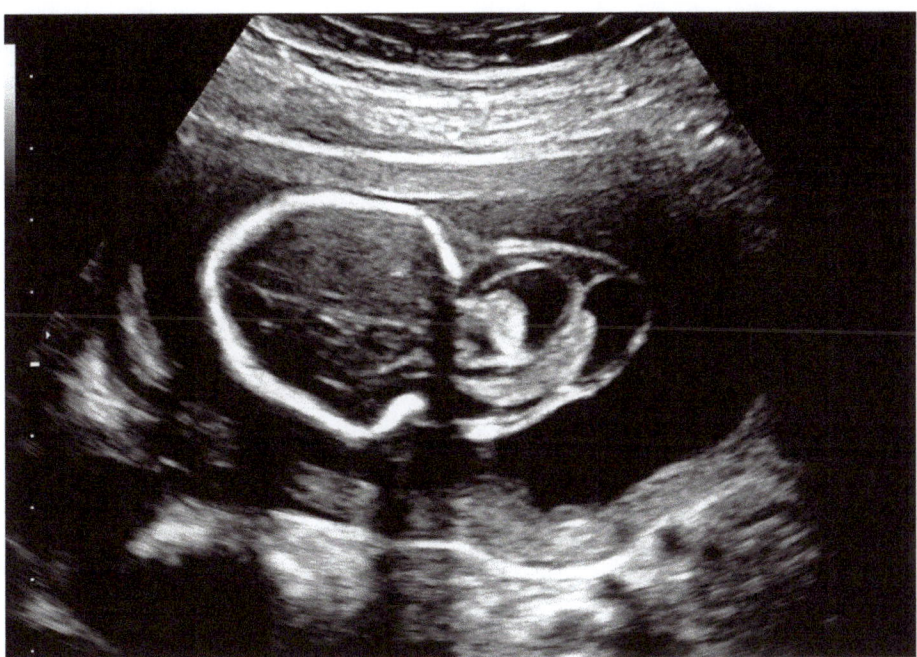

**Fig. 5.21:** B-mode image fetal skull with small bony defect and herniation of the brain—encephalocele.

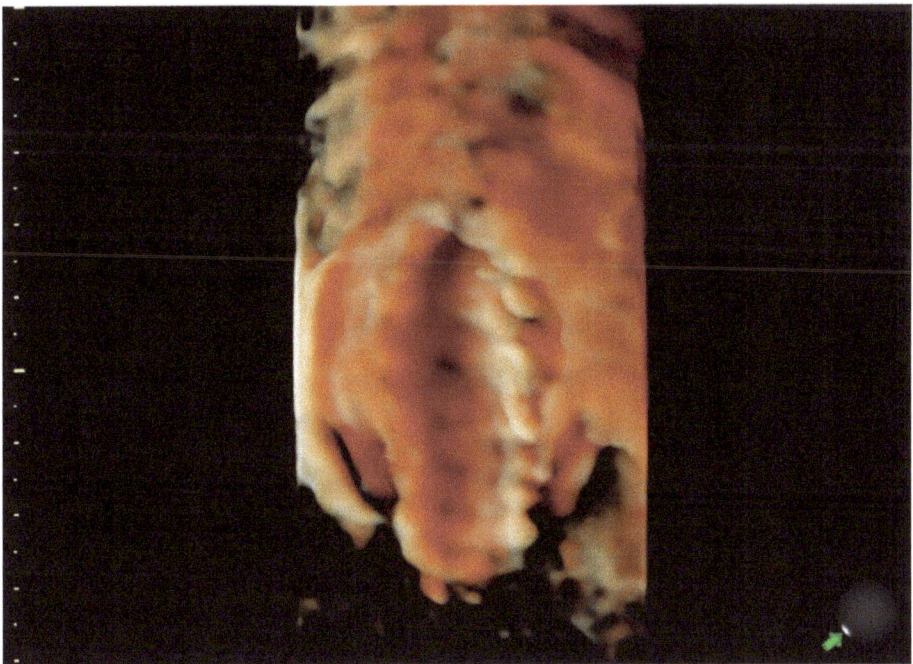

**Fig. 5.22:** Three-dimensional ultrasound rendered image of a large spinal canal defect and also associated large skin defect.

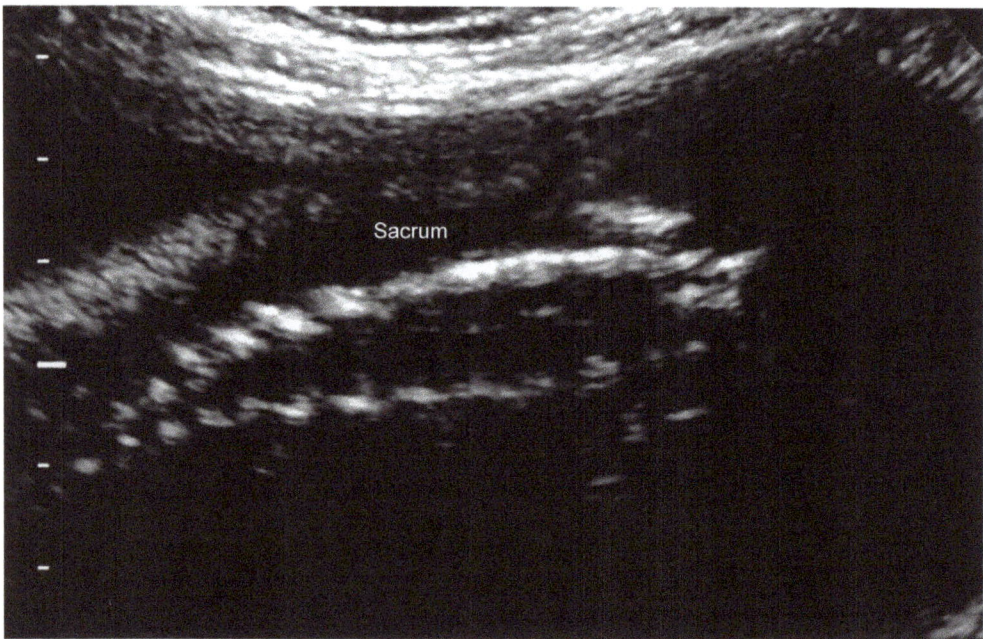

**Fig. 5.23:** B-mode image showing coronal section of the spine with widening of the ossification centers in the lumbar region.

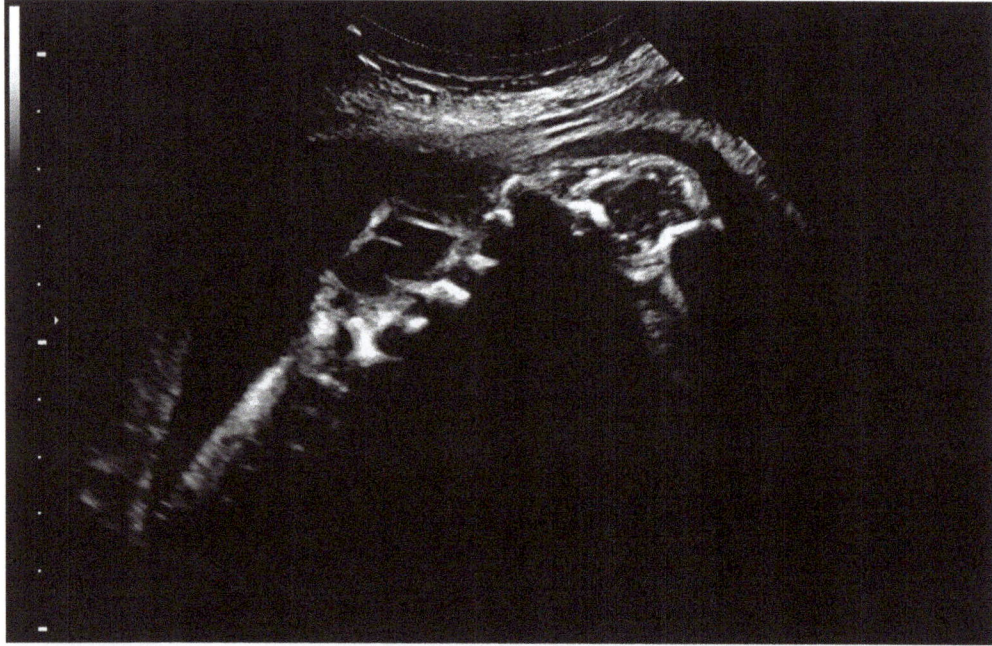

**Fig. 5.24:** B-mode image of sagittal section of spine with abnormal spine contour and a large skin bleb overlying.

## Holoprosencephaly

May be lobar, semilobar or alobar. Alobar is complete absence of falx and non-division of the two cerebral hemispheres and is probably the easiest to diagnose. It is diagnosed on ultrasound by absent falx and cavum septum in axial or coronal sections.

Lobar HPE is the most difficult to diagnose. There is failure of complete separation of the two hemispheres and failure of transverse cleavage into diencephalon and telencephalon. It is the least severe of the classical subtypes of HPE, characterized by the presence of the interhemispheric fissure along almost the entire midline, and with the thalami being completely or nearly completely separated.

On ultrasound lobar HPE shows fusion of the frontal horns of the lateral ventricles, wide communication of the fused segment with the third ventricle, fusion of the fornices, absence of septum pellucidum (Fig. 5.25), normal or hypoplasia of the corpus callosum, anterior cerebral artery may be displaced anteriorly to lie directly underneath the frontal bones (snake under the skull sign).

## Caudal Regression

Caudal regression has the strongest association with diabetes, occurring roughly 200 times more frequently in infants of diabetic mothers than in other infants.[1] Caudal regression is a condition in which there is absent sacrum and variable defects of lumbar spine with agenesis or hypoplasia of the femoral occurs in conjunction and is rare in general population[16] (Fig. 5.26).

This leads to variable degree of motor and neurological defects with incontinence of urine and feces. Apart from the absence of ossification centers of vertebral bodies there are limb defects like club feet and contraction of knees and hips.[62] Approximated or fused iliac wings give a shield-like appearance.

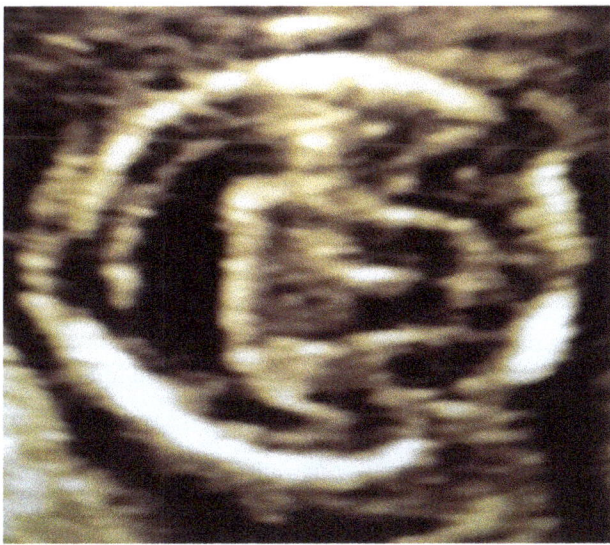

**Fig. 5.25:** B-mode image of the head showing the cranium in the transthallamic section with absent central falx—holoprosencephaly.

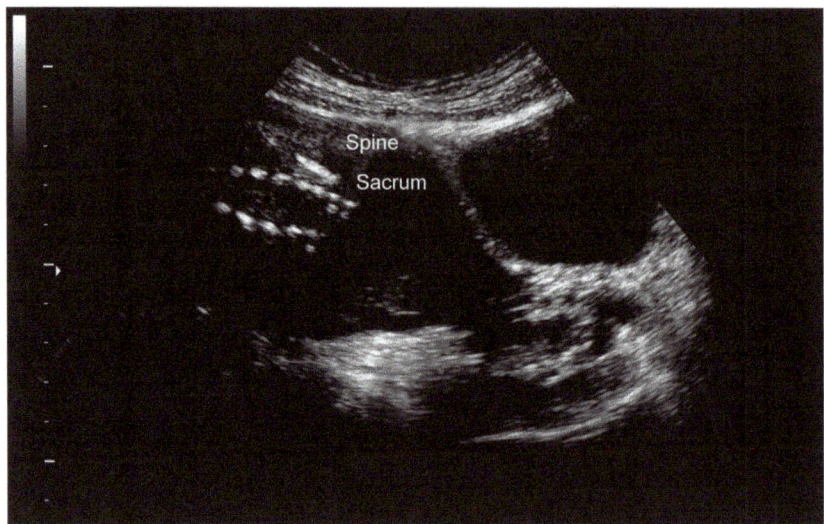

**Fig. 5.26:** B-mode image of the coronal spine with no ossification centers in the sacral area—sacral agenesis.

Decreased interspace between the femoral heads and decreased movements of the legs may also be indicative. Short crown-rump length in the first trimester is indicative of the lesion. It is often associated with other abnormalities involving multiple systems in the fetus.

While the relative risk of caudal regression is many times higher than the relative risk of cardiac anomalies, the magnitude of the problem is actually much greater for cardiac anomalies because their incidence rate is so much higher. One infant in 40 will have congenital heart disease, whereas, even using the highest estimate, only 1 in 350 will have caudal regression.[63]

Median levels of AFP and unconjugated estriol are typically lower in women with pre-existing diabetes, and maternal serum screening programs adjust the marker levels to take account of this difference.[64]

Prognosis depends on severity of spinal defect and associated abnormalities. The recurrence rate is low.

*Sirenomelia* (Fig. 5.27): The diagnostic sign is single lower limb in the midline. It is of course associated with other abnormalities and is lethal.

## Gastrointestinal Tract

These are mostly obstructive—rectal atresia, small left colon. These being obstruction of the distal bowel, the entire small bowel or at least the distal small bowel and large bowel are dilated. The maximum normal diameter of the large bowel in third trimester is 10–12 mm.

### Renal Abnormalities

- Renal agenesis
  *Absence of kidneys*—one or both is known as unilateral or bilateral renal agenesis. It is a routine to document both renal pelvis on a transverse section of the fetal abdomen (Fig. 5.28).

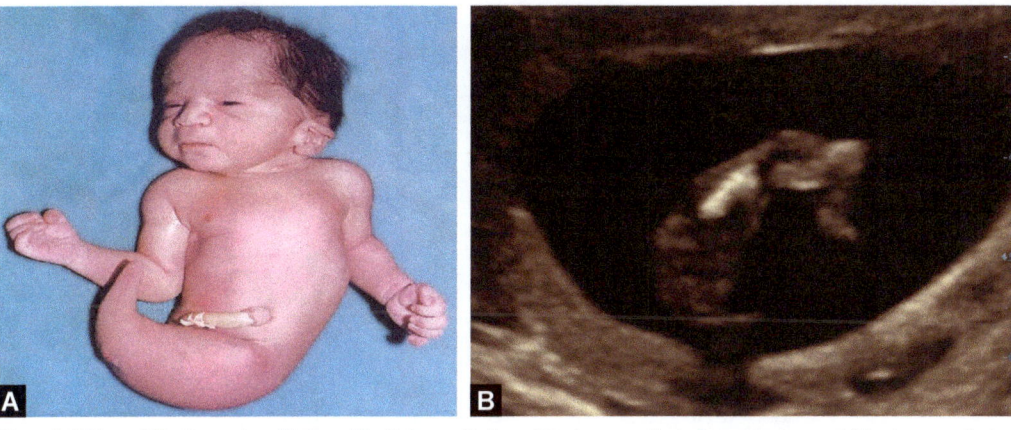

**Figs. 5.27A and B:** Neonate with fused both lower limbs—(A) sirenomelia in fused limbs and (B) sirenomelia in a fetus on ultrasound are shown.

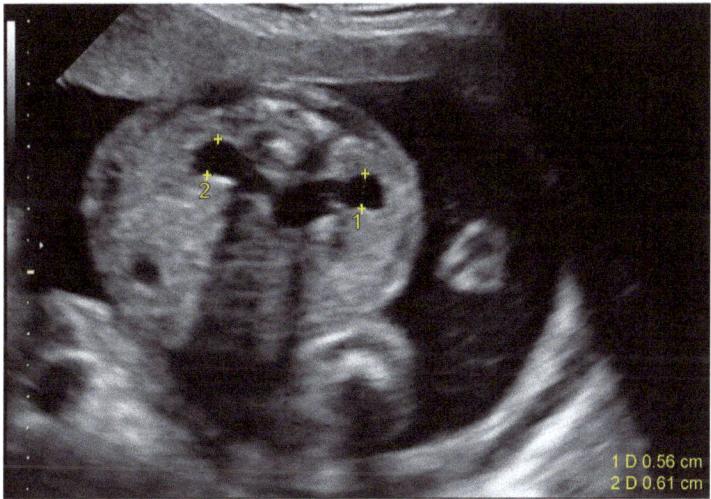

**Fig. 5.28:** Transverse section of the abdomen showing two-renal pelvis as anechoic areas, one on either side of the spine.

Absence of one or both the renal shadows is diagnostic of the condition. Though when the renal shadow is not seen in its usual location, it is important to look for the renal shadow in pelvis or anywhere in the abdomen. For confirmation of the absence of kidney, Doppler can be used. Absence of one or both renal arteries is a supportive and confirmative sign of renal agenesis (Fig. 5.29).

- *Hydronephrosis*: Normal renal pelvis diameter in axial section is 4 mm at 16–20 weeks, 5 mm at 20–30 weeks, and 7 mm at 30–40 weeks. Anything more than these measurements is considered as renal pyelectasis. But for correct diagnosis it is important that the axial section of the renal pelvis in true axial, bilateral symmetrical, stomach shadow or bladder

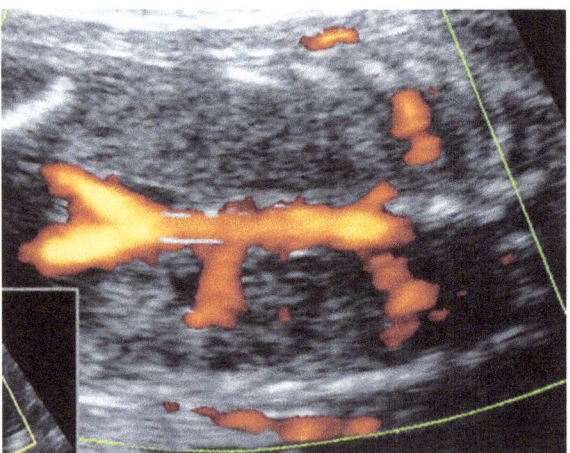

**Fig. 5.29:** Coronal section of the fetal abdomen with power Doppler showing aorta and only one renal artery suggestive of agenesis of one of the kidneys.

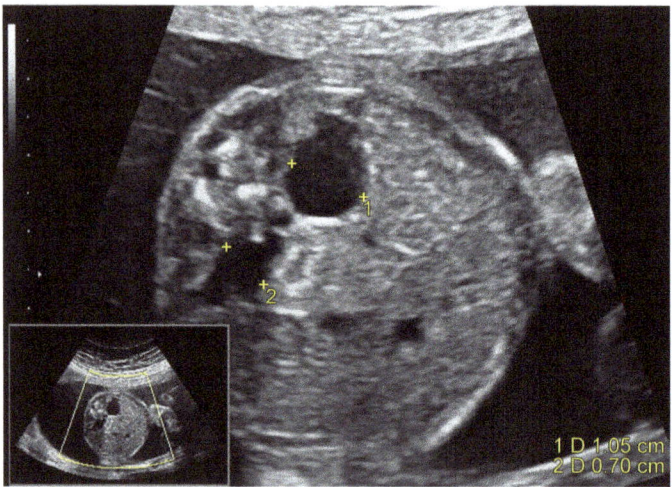

**Fig. 5.30:** Transverse section of fetal abdomen, showing bilateral dilated renal pelvis, one side being more dilated than the other.

should not be seen on this plane and diameter is measured inner to inner margin of renal pelvis in anteroposterior direction (Fig. 5.30). But it is important to differentiate renal pyelectasis from hydronephrosis. Hydronephrosis is confirmed by dilatation of the entire pelvicalyceal system (Fig. 5.31).

- *Ureteric duplication*: This is difficult to diagnose antenatally, unless there is dilatation of both the ureters (Fig. 5.32).
- *Multicystic dysplasia*: Renal dysplasias found in fetuses of diabetic mothers are more nonobstructive. These may be microcystic or macrocystic. Microcystic renal dysplasias show hyperechoic kidneys (Fig. 5.33) and macrocystic renal dysplasia shows multiple anechoic areas in the kidneys which are cysts (Fig. 5.34).

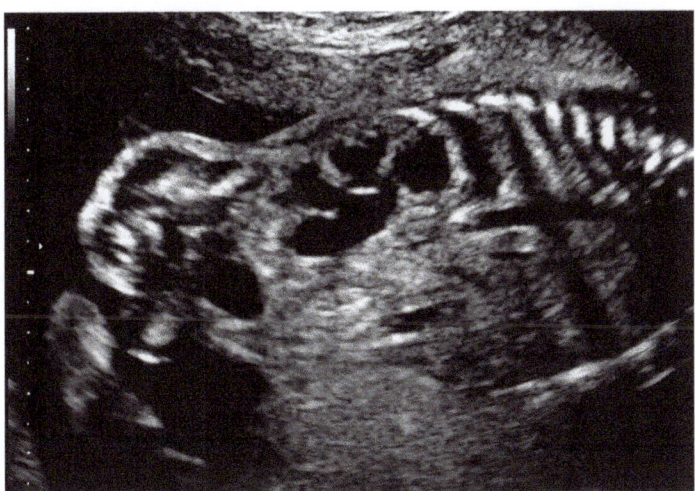

**Fig. 5.31:** On sagittal section of the fetus on B-mode ultrasound showing dilated renal pelvicalyceal system.

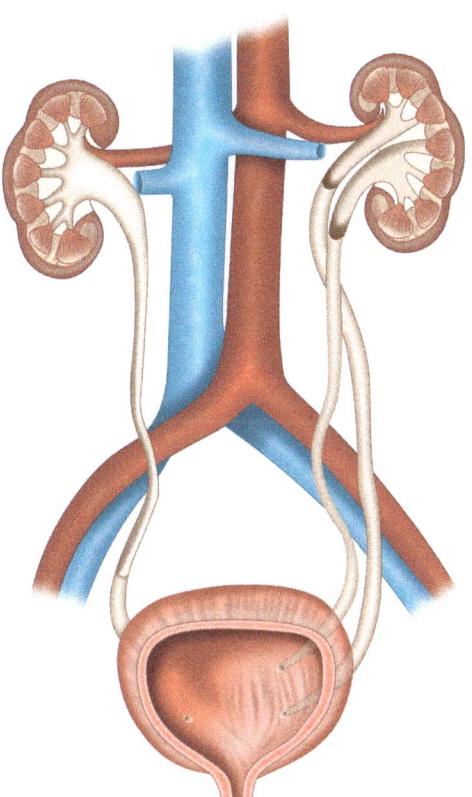

**Fig. 5.32:** Diagrammatic representation of double ureter on left side. Though this is difficult to diagnose on antenatal scan without dilatation of the pelvicalyceal system and ureter.

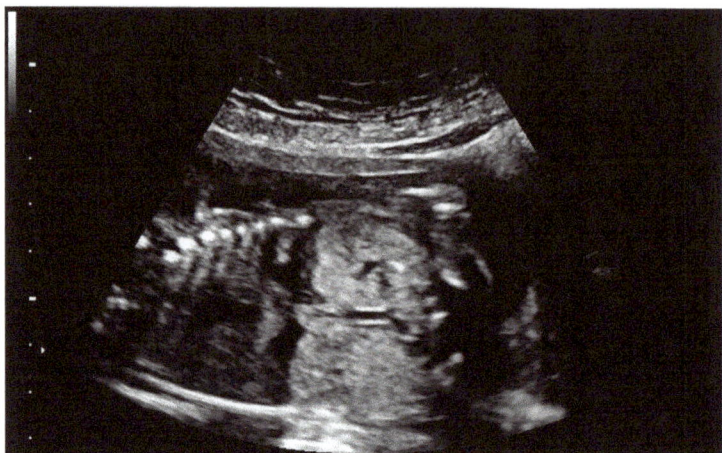

**Fig. 5.33:** Coronal plane image of the fetus on B-mode ultrasound showing hyperechoic kidneys—microcystic renal dysplasia.

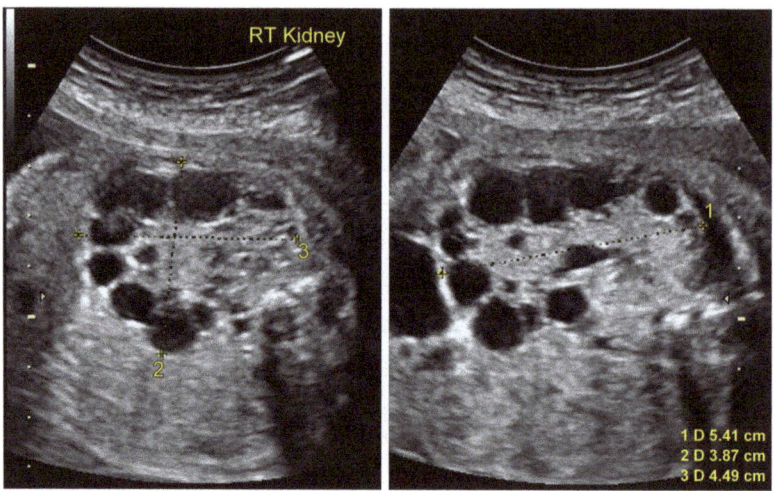

**Fig. 5.34:** B-mode ultrasound of the fetus showing multiple anechoic cystic areas in the kidney suggesting macrocystic dysplastic kidney.

## Skeletal Abnormalities

Polydactyly, syndactyly (Figs. 5.35A and B), and short femur are all signs of different chromosomal abnormalities. Therefore, whenever these are found it is very important to make an intense search for any associated abnormalities by a detailed ultrasound scan.

## Macrosomia and Polyhydramnios

Macrosomia or large for gestational age is defined as a fetus with estimated weight of more than 90th percentile. Roughly this estimates to the birth weight at term of more than 4,500 g. Incidence of macrosomia in fetuses of diabetic mothers is 17–50%.

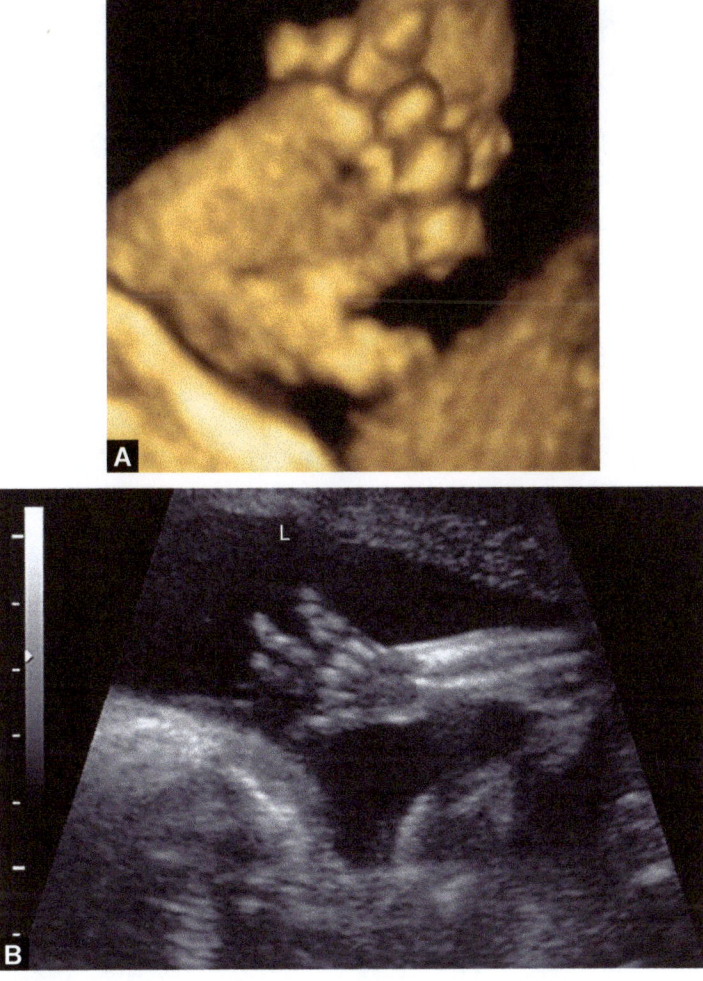

**Figs. 5.35A and B:** (A) Three-dimensional ultrasound image showing polydactyly; (B) B-mode image of the fetal hand showing the last two fingers joined with each other—syndactyly.

Macrosomia can be assessed by weight or by biometry. The most commonly used biometric parameters are abdominal circumference (AC) and femur length (FL) in combination. As these are diagnostic criteria, it is important to follow standard sections of fetal abdomen and femur and standardized measuring technique.

The AC is measured on the transverse section of the abdomen that cuts through the stomach and shows the middle third of the umbilical vein taking a curve towards right side, forming a "J" shape, to continue to feed the liver (Fig. 5.36). The section should be round and bilateral symmetrical ribs should be seen. The circumference is drawn on the outer margin of the circumference. Femur is measured from proximal end of the diaphysis to the distal end of the diaphysis (Fig. 5.37). The section is obtained in such a way that the lateral lobe artifact does not distort the ends of the bones, as this may lead to erroneous assessment of the FL. AC less

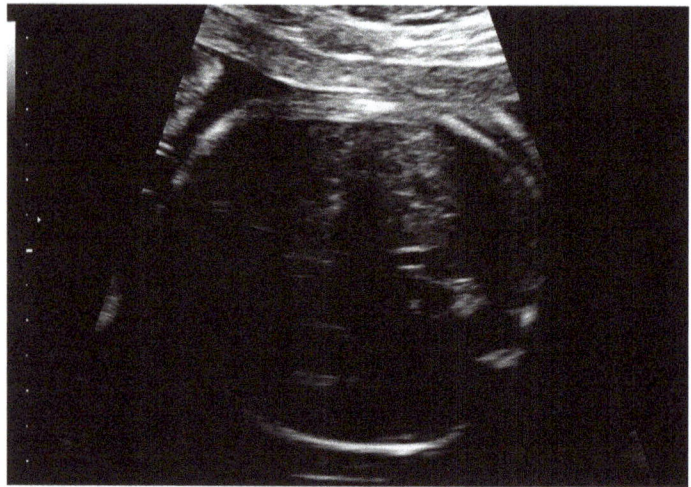

**Fig. 5.36:** B-mode ultrasound image of the transverse section of the abdomen.

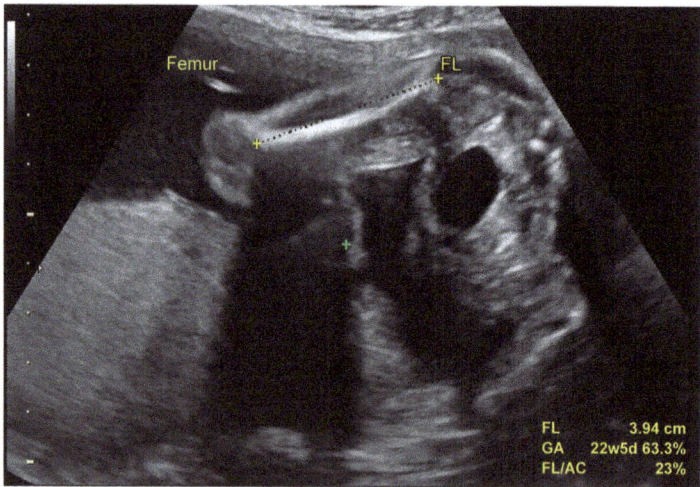

**Fig. 5.37:** B-mode ultrasound image of the femur.

than 35 cm reduces the risk of baby being more than 4,500 g to as low as 1%.[65] But if AC is more than 38 cm, the risk of birth weight being more than 4,500 g is 37%.

But diagnosis of macrosomia is not reliable and 90% of these babies have no complications. More sophisticatedly it can be diagnosed by assessment of body fat at the mid upper arm, mid-thigh or abdominal subcutaneous fat.[14] The major risk of macrosomia is shoulder dystocia and intrapartum complications.

It is commonly associated with polyhydramnios. As shown in different studies 27–37% prevalence of macrosomia is seen in pregnancies with polyhydramnios. The risk of macrosomia is increased to as much as 2.7-fold in presence of polyhydramnios.[66,67]

Polyhydramnios is also more common in fetuses of diabetic mothers. The association is probably thought to be due to:

- Increased renal vascular flow
- Reversal of intermembranous flow (from fetal circulation to amniotic fluid)
- Increase in the volume of fluid excreted by the fetal lungs.

With polyhydramnios, early labor and prematurity is a major problem.

Prematurity carries its own complications and high neonatal morbidity and mortality. Though it is interesting to know that even in absence of polyhydramnios, preterm delivery is a known complication of diabetes (IDDM) itself. Though its incidence is lower in patients with gestational diabetes.[68]

Recurrent polyhydramnios in subsequent pregnancy is seen only in about 5% of cases, but in those in whom recurrent polyhydramnios is seen, 25% are diabetic.

## Ultrasound Assessment of Polyhydramnios

In third trimester, transverse section of the abdomen of the fetus almost extends from anterior to posterior wall of the uterus. Fluid seen therefore around the fetal abdomen is a subjective sign of polyhydramnios in the third trimester (Fig. 5.38).

Though semiquantitative assessment is more accurate. The amniotic fluid conventionally was measured as the largest pocket of fluid in four quadrants of the uterus, assessed with the probe vertically placed on the maternal abdomen. The pocket should be devoid of cord loops or limbs. The measurement is the vertical largest diameter of each pocket (Fig. 5.39). Amniotic fluid index is calculated as total of these four distances. The total of more than 20 cm is mild, more than 24 cm is moderate, and more than 25 cm is severe polyhydramnios.[69,70] The latter is more commonly associated with macrosomia.

Though according to the more recent trend, amniotic fluid is calculated as the largest vertical diameter of the largest fluid pocket. This measurement of more than 8 cm is mild, more than 12 cm is moderate, and more than 16 cm is severe polyhydramnios.[71]

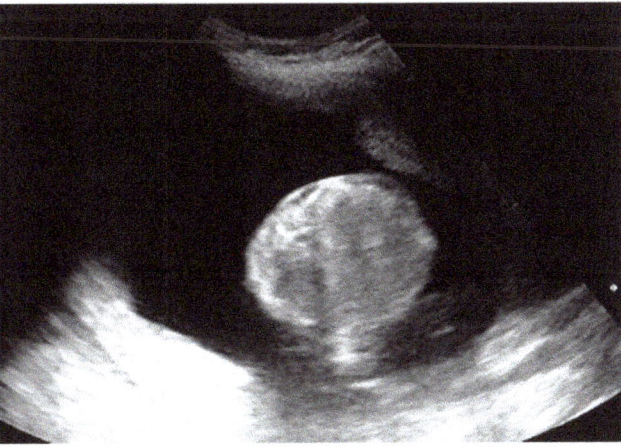

**Fig. 5.38:** B-mode ultrasound image of the fetal abdomen in transverse section with amniotic fluid all around suggestive of polyhydramnios.

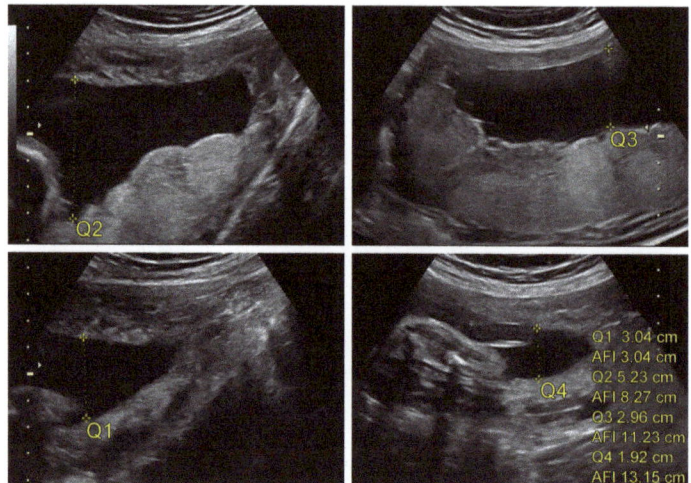

**Fig. 5.39:** B-mode ultrasound images in quadruple frame usually taken for assessment of amniotic fluid index.

Indomethacin is an effective drug for the treatment of diabetes-related polyhydramnios. It is given as 25 mg every 6 hours and has shown to decrease the amniotic fluid volume as early as 21 weeks.[72] But carries a risk of several maternal and fetal complications. Of the fetal complications majority are related to early closure of ductus arteriosus that it causes, leading to pulmonary hypertension, intraventricular hemorrhage, necrotizing enterocolitis and in severe cases may also lead to fetal death.

## CONCLUSION

Diabetes in pregnancy is of major concern for fetal health. It is associated with several abnormalities involving almost all different body systems of the fetus. The abnormalities are associated more with type I diabetes rather than gestational diabetes. But it is also important to note that the incidence of abnormalities is significantly decreased in pregnancies with good glycemic control, especially since conception. It is therefore very important to investigate for diabetes or insulin resistance in all the pregnancy-desiring females, and treat them. Their close follow-up and perfect glycemic control may be possibly the best strategy to control diabetes-associated fetal malformations.

## REFERENCES

1. Mills JL. Malformations in infants of diabetic mothers. Birth Defects Res A Clin Mol Teratol. 2010;88(10):769-78.
2. Eskes TK, Mooij PN, Steegers-Theunissen RP, et al. Pregnancy care and prevention of birth defects. J Perinat Med. 1992;20(4):253-65.
3. Goto MP, Goldman AS. Diabetic embryopathy. Curr Opin Ped. 1994;6:486-91.
4. Hod M, Diamant YZ. The offspring of a diabetic mother-short and long range implications. Israel J Med Sci. 1992;28(2):81-6.
5. Miller E, Hare JW, Cloherty JP, et al. Elevated maternal hemoglobin Alc in early pregnancy and major congenital anomalies in infants of diabetic mothers. N Engl J Med. 1981;304:1331-4.

6. Mills JL, Baker L, Goldman AS. Malformations of infants of diabetic mothers occur before the 7th gestational week: Implications for treatment. Diabetes. 1979;28(4):292-3.
7. Mills JL. Malformations in infants of diabetic mothers. Teratology. 1982;25(3):385-94.
8. Mills JL, Knopp RH, Simpson JL, et al. NIHHD and diabetes in early pregnancy study: lack of relation of increased malformation rates in infants of diabetic mothers to glycemic control during organogenesis. N Engl J Med. 1991;318:671-6.
9. Miodovnik M, Mimouni F, Dignan PS, et al. Major malformations in infants of IDDM women: Vasculopathy and early first-trimester poor glycemic control. Diabetes Care. 1988;11(9):713-8.
10. Miller E, Hare JW, Cloherty JP, et al. Elevated maternal hemoglobin Alc in early pregnancy and major congenital anomalies in infants of diabetic mothers. N Engl J Med. 1981;304:1331-4.
11. Blumenthal SA, Abdul-Karim W. Diagnosis, classifications, and metabolic management of diabetes in pregnancy: therapeutic impact of self-monitoring of blood glucose and of newer methods of insulin delivery. Obstet Gynecol Surveys. 1987;42:593-603.
12. Cordero L, London MB. Infants of the diabetic mother. Clin Perinatol. 1993;20(3):635-48.
13. Leslie RD, Pyke DA, John PN, et al. Hemoglobin Alc in diabetic pregnancy. Lancet. 1978;ii: 958-62.
14. Evers IM, de Valk HW, Visser GH. Risk of complications of pregnancy in women with type I diabetes: Nationwide prospective study in the Netherlands. Br Med J. 2004;328(7445):915-20.
15. Pedersen LM, Tygstrup I, Pedersen J. Congenital malformations in newborn infants of diabetic women. Lancet. 1964;1(7343):1124-6.
16. Kucera J. Rate and type of congenital anomalies among offspring of diabetic women. J Reprod Med. 1971;7(2):73-82.
17. Churchill JA, Berendes HW, Nemore J. Neuropsychological deficits in children of diabetic mothers: a report from the collaborative study of cerebral palsy. Am J Obstet Gynecol. 1969;105(2): 257-68.
18. Day RE, Insley J. Maternal diabetes mellitus and congenital malformation. Survey of 205 cases. Arch Dis Child. 1976;51(12):935-8.
19. Ramos-Arroyo MA, Rodriguez-Pinilla E, Cordero JF. Maternal diabetes: the risk for specific birth defects. Eur J Epidemiol. 1992;8(4):503-8.
20. Anderson JL, Waller DK, Canfield MA, et al. Maternal obesity, gestational diabetes, and central nervous system birth defects. Epidemiology. 2005;16(1):87-92.
21. Meltzer SJ, Ryan EA, Feig DS, et al. Preconception care for women with diabetes. Canadian Diabetes Association, Clinical Practice Guidelines, 2003.
22. Langer O, Conway DL. Level of glycemia and perinatal outcome in pregestational diabetes. J Matern Fetal Med. 2000;9(1):35-41.
23. American Diabetes Association. Gestational diabetes mellitus. Diabetes Care. 2000;23 Suppl 1:S77-9.
24. Temple R, Aldridge V, Greenwood R, et al. Association between outcome of pregnancy in type 1 diabetes: population based study. BMJ. 2002;325(7375):1275-6.
25. The Diabetes Control Complications Trial Research Group. Pregnancy outcomes in the Diabetes Control and Complications trial. Am J Obstet Gynecol. 1996;174:1343-53.
26. Schaefer-Graf UM, Buchanan TA, Xiang A, et al. Patterns of congenital anomalies and relationship to initial maternal fasting glucose levels in pregnancies complicated by type 2 and gestational diabetes. Am J Obstet Gynecol. 2000;182(2):313-20.
27. Suhonen L, Hiilesmaa V, Teramo K. Glycaemic control during early pregnancy and fetal malformations in women with type 1 diabetes mellitus. Diabetologia. 2000;43(1):79-82.
28. Hanson U, Persson B, Thunell S. Relationship between haemoglobin A1C in early type 1 (insulin-dependent) diabetic pregnancy and the occurrence of spontaneous abortion and fetal malformation in Sweden. Diabetologia. 1990;33(2):100-4.
29. Farrell T, Neale L, Cundy T. Congenital anomalies in the offspring of women with type 1, type 2 and gestational diabetes. Diabet Med. 2002;19(4):322-6.

30. McElduff A. Cheung NW, McIntyre HD, et al. The Australasian Diabetes in Pregnancy Society consensus guidelines for the management of type 1 and type 2 diabetes in relation to pregnancy. Med J Aust. 2005;183(7):373-7.
31. The Diabetes Control Complications Trial Research Group. Pregnancy outcomes in the Diabetes Control and Complications trial. Am J Obstet Gynecol. 1996;174(4):1343-53.
32. Sharpe PB, Chan A, Haan EA, et al. Maternal diabetes and congenital anomalies in South Australia 1986–2000: a population-based cohort study. Birth Defects Res A Clin Mol Teratol. 2005;73(9):605-11.
33. Martinez-Frias ML, Bermejo E, Rodriguez-Pinilla E, et al. Epidemiological analysis of outcomes of pregnancy in gestational diabetic mothers. Am J Med Genetics. 1998;78(2):140-5.
34. Versiani BR, Gilbert-Barness E, Giuliani LR, et al. Caudal dysplasia sequence: severe phenotype presenting in offspring of patients with gestational and pregestational diabetes. Clin Dysmorphol. 2004;13(1):1-5.
35. Soler NG. Perinatal Medicine. Fifth European Congress of Perinatology. Stockholm: Almqvist and Wiksell Int; 1976.
36. Soler N, Walsh C, Malins JM. Congenital malformations in newborn infants of diabetic mothers. Q J Med. 1976;178:303-13.
37. Chung CS, Myrianthopoulos NC. Factors affecting risks of congenital malformations. II. Effect of maternal diabetes on congenital malformations. Birth Defects Orig Artic Ser. 1975;11(10):23-38.
38. Pedersen JF, Sorenson S, Molsted-Pederson L. Pregnancy associated plasma protein A in first trimester of diabetiec pregnancy and subsequent fetal growth. Acta Obstet Gynecol Scand. 1998;77(9):932-4.
39. Ong CY, Liao AW, Spencer K, et al. First trimester maternal serum free-hCG and PAPP-A as predictors of pregnancy complications. Br J Obstet Gynecol. 2000;107:1265-70.
40. Palomaki GE, Knight GJ, Haddow JE. Human chorionic gonadotrophin and unconjugated oestriol measurements in insulin dependent diabetic pregnancy women being screened for fetal Down syndrome. Prenat Diagn. 1994;14(1):65-8.
41. Kousseff BG. Diabetic embryopathy. Curr Opin Pediatr. 1999;11(4):348.
42. Aberg A, Westbom L, Kallen B. Congenital malformations among infants whose mothers had gestational diabetes or pre-existing diabetes. Early Hum Dev. 2001;61(2):85-95.
43. Sheffield JS, Butler-Koster EL, Casey BM, et al. Maternal diabetes and infant malformations. Obstet Gynecol. 2002;100(5 Pt 1):925-30.
44. Chh-Ping Chen. Congenital malformaltions associated with maternal diabetes. Taiwanese Journal of Obstetrics and Gynecology. 2005;44(1):1-7.
45. Wang R, Martinez-Frias ML, Graham JM Jr. Infants of diabetic mothers are at increased risk for the oculo-auriculo-vertebral sequence: a case-based and case-control approach. J Pediatr. 2002;141(5):611-7.
46. Meyer-Wittkopf M, Simpson JM, Sharland GK. Incidence of congenital heart defects in fetuses of diabetic mothers: a retrospective study of 326 cases. Ultrasound Obstet Gynecol. 1996;8(1):8-10.
47. Wheller JJ, Reiss R, Allen HD. Clinical experience with fetal echocardiography. Am J Dis Child. 1990;144(1):49-53.
48. Zielinsky P. Role of prenatal echocardiography in the study of hypertrophic cardiomyopathy in the fetus. Echocardiography. 1991;8(6):661-8.
49. Cooper MJ, Enderlein MA, Dyson DC, et al. Fetal echocardiography: retrospective review of clinical experience and an evaluation of indications. Obstet Gynecol. 1995;86(4 Pt 1):577-82.
50. Buskens E, Stewart PA, Hess J, et al. Efficacy of fetal echocardiography and yield by risk category. Obstet Gynecol. 1996;87(3):423-8.
51. Adams MM, Mulinare J, Dooley K. Risk factors for conotruncal cardiac defects in Atlanta. J Am Coll Cardiol. 1989;14(2):432-42.
52. Ferencz C, Rubin JD, McCarter RJ, et al. Maternal diabetes and cardiovascular malformations: predominance of double outlet right ventricle and truncus arteriosus. Teratology. 1990;41(3):319-26.

53. Mace S, Hirschfield SS, Riggs T, et al. Echocardiographic abnormalities in infants of diabetic mothers. J Pediatr. 1979;95(6):1013-9.
54. Seppanen MP, Ojanpera OS, Kaapa PO, et al. Delayed postnatal adaptation of pulmonary hemodynamics in infants of diabetic mothers. J Pediatr. 1997;131(4):545-8.
55. Vural M, Leke L, Mahomedaly H, et al. Should an echocardiographic scan be done routinely for infants of diabetic mothers? Turk J Pediatr. 1995;37(4):351-6.
56. Walther FJ, Siassi B, King J, et al. Cardiac output in infants of insulin-dependent diabetic mothers. J Pediatr. 1985;107(1):109-14.
57. Gutgesell HP, Mullins CE, Gillette PC, et al. Transient hypertrophic subaortic stenosis in infants of diabetic mothers. J Pediatr. 1976;89(1):120-5.
58. Halliday HL. Hypertrophic cardiomyopathy in infants of poorly-controlled diabetic mothers. Arch Dis Child. 1981;56(4):258-63.
59. Rizzo G, Arduini D, Romanini C. Accelerated cardiac growth and abnormal cardiac flow in fetuses of type I diabetic mothers. Am J Obstet Gynecol. 1991;164(3):837-43.
60. Fenichel P, Hieronimus S, Bourlon F, et al. Macrosomie du foetus de mère diabétique. Presse Med. 1990;19(6):255-8.
61. Way GL, Wolfe RR, Eshaghpour E, et al. The natural history of hypertrophic cardiomyopathy in infants of diabetic mothers. J Pediatr. 1979;95(6):1020-5.
62. Benacerraf BR. Caudal Regression Syndrome and Sirenomelia in Ultrasound of Fetal Syndromes. New York: Churchill Livingstone; 1998. pp. 250-4.
63. Pedersen J. The Pregnant Diabetic and Her Newborn. Copenhagen: Munksgaard; 1977. p. 194.
64. Martinez-Frias ML, Frias JP, Bermejo E, et al. Pre-gestational maternal body mass index predicts an increased risk of congenital malformations in infants of mothers with gestational diabetes. Diabet Med. 2005;22(6):775-81.
65. Gilby JR, Williams MC, Spellacy WN. Fetal abdominal circumference measurements of 35 and 38 cm as predictors of macrosomia. A risk factor for shoulder dystocia. J Reprod Med. 2000;45(11):936-8.
66. Sohaey R, Nyberg D, Sickler GK, et al. Idiopathic polyhydramnios: association with fetal macrosomia. Radiology. 1994;190(2):393-6.
67. Lazebnik N, Hill LM, Guzick D, et al. Severity of polyhydramnios does not affect the prevalence of large for gestational age new born infants. J Ultrasound Med. 1996;15:385-8.
68. Many A, Hill LM, Lazebnik N, et al. The association between polyhydramnios and preterm delivery. Obstet Gynecol. 1995;86(3):389-91.
69. Smith CV, Plambeck RD, Rayburn WF, et al. Relation of mild idiopathic polyhydramnios to perinatal outcome. Obstet Gynecol. 1992;79(3):387-9.
70. Biggio JR, Wenstrom KD, Dubard MB, et al. Hydramnios prediction of adverse perinatal outcome. Obstet Gynecol. 1999;94(5 Pt 1):773-7.
71. Hill LM, Breckle R, Thomas ML, et al. Polyhydramnios: ultrasonically detected prevalence and neonatal outcome. Obstet Gynecol. 1987;69(1):21-5.
72. Mamopoulos M, Assimakopoulas E, Reece EA, et al. Maternal indomethacin therapy in the treatment of polyhydramnios. Am J Obstet Gynecol. 1990;162(5):1225-9.

# Chapter 6

# Obstetric Ultrasound for Diabetes-related Congenital Anomalies

*Karim D Kalache, Farhat Gothey, Alexander Weichert, Daniel Kamil*

## PREGESTATIONAL AND GESTATIONAL DIABETES AND THE RISK OF MAJOR CONGENITAL ANOMALIES

Diabetes is the most common medical complication in pregnancy. Women with diabetes in pregnancy can be divided into two groups: pregestational diabetes which complicates less than 1% of all pregnancies is defined as type 1 (previously referred to as insulin-dependent diabetes mellitus or juvenile-onset diabetes mellitus) or type 2 diabetes (previously referred to as non-insulin-dependent diabetes mellitus or adult-onset diabetes mellitus) that exists before the pregnancy. In about 2% of all pregnancies, the glucose intolerance is first diagnosed during pregnancy and is termed gestational diabetes. Gestational diabetes is further subdivided according to the degree of severity of the glycemic control disturbance. Women with normal fasting plasma glucose are referred to as Class A and those with abnormal fasting plasma glucose are categorized as Class B. "Underutilization" constitutes the principal metabolic disturbance in Class A, whereas Class B are experiencing varying degrees of "increased production" in addition to "reduced utilization" and might in reality represent undiagnosed pregestational diabetes type 2.

The risk of major congenital malformations is significantly higher in women with pregestational diabetes mellitus,[1] especially when glycemia is not well controlled during the periconceptional period.[2] Whether the risk of major congenital anomalies is also higher in gestational diabetes mellitus is still the subject of a debate. Some authors[3,4] have reported that there is an increased risk of congenital anomalies in the offspring of a diabetic mother, while others[2,5] have reported a risk that is similar to the reference group except for women with Class B gestational diabetes.[2] Difficulties in the definition of gestational diabetes and the fact that gestational diabetes does not distinguish between unrecognized type 2 diabetes and glucose intolerance caused by the hormonal-related pregnancy changes might explain the ongoing discussion about the association between major congenital anomalies and gestational diabetes.

## INCIDENCE AND IMPACT OF CONGENITAL ANOMALIES

It is reported that in the offspring of women with pregestational diabetes, the risk of congenital anomalies is increased by five when compared with the general population.[6] The two fetal organ that are most frequently affected are the fetal heart with the incidence of cardiovascular abnormalities ranging from 0.2% to 3% and the central nervous system with the incidence of central nervous system abnormalities ranging from 0.1% to 5%.[2] Other organ systems that are frequently affected are the musculoskeletal (abnormalities from 0.2% to 2%) and the genitourinary system (abnormalities from 0.2% to 3%).[2] The link between hyperglycemia and congenital anomalies has been established, but the precise mechanism it occurs has not been completely elaborated. It is recognized that even minimal deviations in glucose levels could be dangerous for the developing embryo.[7,8] While enhanced specialized antenatal care has considerably reduced the frequency of diabetes-related intrauterine fetal death, major congenital anomalies are still the cause of the majority of perinatal deaths among infants of diabetic mothers.[9] It is well recognized that major congenital anomalies are the cause of about 25% of the perinatal deaths associated with diabetic pregnancies.

## CAUDAL REGRESSION SYNDROME

Caudal regression syndrome (also frequently referred to as sacral dys- or agenesis, caudal dysplasia or phocomelic diabetic embryopathy) is characterized by abnormal formation of the distal spine and pelvis. It is the only abnormality that is known to be specifically associated and typical for diabetes in pregnancy. Animal experiments conducted in the early 50s found that insulin administration into the yolk sac of chicken embryos was frequently associated with caudal anomalies consisting of either partial or total absence of tail structures. The most accepted explanation for this syndrome is failure of induction of the caudal elements before the 7th week of gestation.

Given the interdependency of neighboring structures on the caudal elements an entire range of congenital malformations (Table 6.1) affecting the caudal region of the fetus can also be seen as part of this condition. Caudal regression syndrome can be seen sporadically, but it is 200 times more common in offsprings of diabetic mothers. The incidence of this congenital anomaly in the normal population is about 1 per 25,000 live births and is about 150–200 times more common in infants of diabetic mothers.[10-13]

Imaging of the spine is usually easily achieved when the fetus is in a dorso-anterior position with enough amniotic fluid above it (Fig. 6.1). The fetal thoracolumbar spine curvature has a "c" shape with sacral "tapering" which should be seen in all fetuses after

| Table 6.1: Characteristic elements of caudal regression syndrome. | |
|---|---|
| Anomalies of the lower extremities | Bilateral femoral hypoplasia Unilateral femoral hypoplasia |
| Vertebral anomalies | Sacral agenesis Spina bifida |
| Gastrointestinal tract | Anal atresia |
| Urinary tract | Renal agenesis Urethral agenesis Bilateral pelvic kidneys |
| Genital anomalies | Cloacal anomaly Hydrometrocolpos Cryptorchidism Hypospadia |

22 weeks of gestation. Prenatal diagnosis of caudal regression syndrome by ultrasound is possible by showing as sudden interruption of the spine with absent "tapering" due to absence of lower vertebrae (Figs. 6.2 and 6.3). The position of the conus medullaris in relation to the spine changes with advancing gestational age as the spine develops and grows faster than the spinal cord. Its position is most frequently between L2 and L3 between 19 weeks' gestation and 24 weeks' gestation (Fig. 6.4). Then, it undergoes its progressive relative ascent to be located above L2–L3 at term. The conus medullaris in caudal regression syndrome is abnormally high. Absent pelvic bones can be challenging to demonstrate.

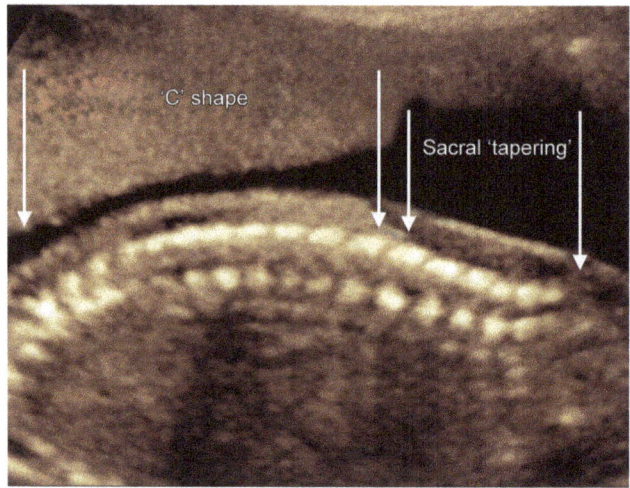

**Fig. 6.1:** Normal fetal spine at 22 weeks gestation with "C" shaped curvature with sacral "tapering".

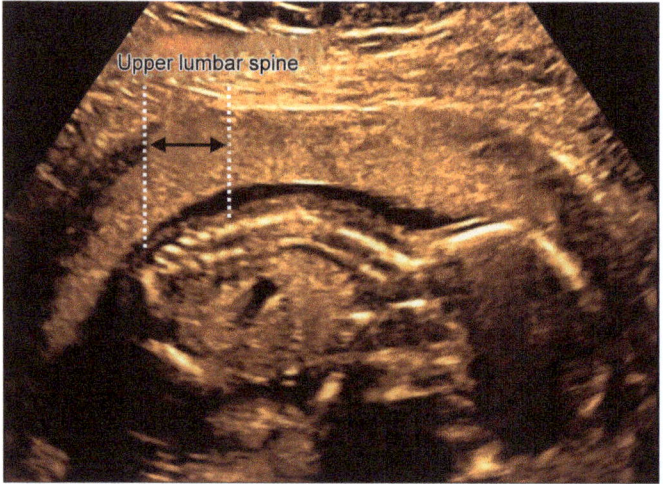

**Fig. 6.2:** Caudal regression syndrome at 16 weeks gestational age. There is a shortened spine with absence of sacral "tapering".

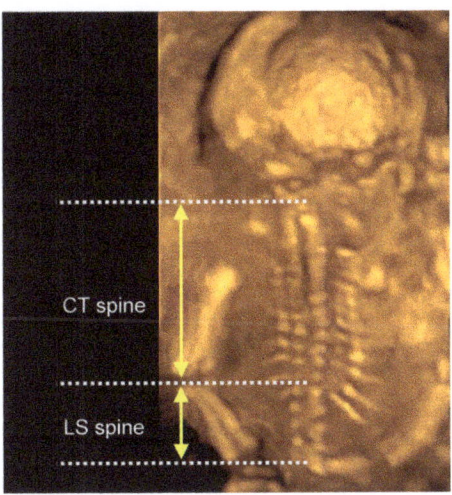

**Fig. 6.3:** Caudal regression syndrome at 16 weeks gestational age on 3D maximum rendering mode. Note the shortened lumbosacral (LS) spine when compared with cervicothoracic (CT) spine.

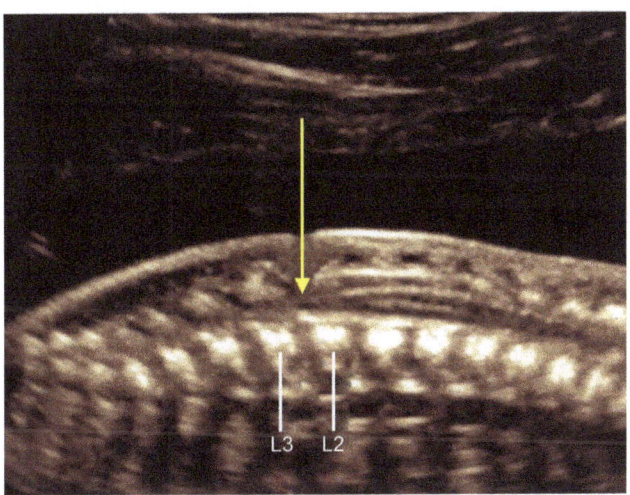

**Fig. 6.4:** Normal fetal spine at 22 weeks gestation with the level of the conus medullaris (arrow) between L3 and L2.

With the advent of first trimester screening, the fetal anatomy can be studied as early as 12 weeks of gestation. Caudal regression syndrome is anatomically present in the first trimester, but will go undetected if the focus and interest is on the nuchal translucency and the gestational age is wrongly corrected as affected fetuses will have an abnormally small crown rump length.

## STRUCTURAL CARDIAC DEFECTS AND CARDIAC ANOMALIES

Children of diabetic mothers are much more likely to have congenital heart defects. Moreover, congenital heart defects are among the most important causes of perinatal mortality in offspring of diabetic mothers.[14-21] A large Canadian study based on the assessment of congenital anomalies among nearly 2 million children, observed a 47% higher prevalence of congenital abnormalities overall and up to a three- to fivefold higher prevalence of various cardiac anomalies among newborns of mothers with diabetes compared with those born to mothers without diabetes.[22]

The association between maternal diabetes mellitus and congenital cardiac abnormalities has been recognized for more than 50 years. The most common cardiac anomalies associated with diabetes in pregnancy are transposition of the great vessels, common arterial trunk, ventricular septal defects, visceral heterotaxia, and coarctation of the aorta,[23,24] suggesting teratogenesis during cardiac looping and/or conotruncal septation.

Transposition of the great arteries is a conotruncal abnormality in which the right heart receiving blood body ejects blood directly in the aorta and the left heart receiving blood from the lungs ejects blood directly into the pulmonary artery. In other words, the aorta arises from the right ventricle and the pulmonary artery arises from the left ventricle. Transposition of the great arteries is a common form of cyanotic congenital heart disease and one in which prenatal diagnosis has an important impact on neonatal outcomes.

The outflow tract assessment is important for the diagnosis of transposition of the great arteries. Characteristic ultrasound images in D-transposition of the great arteries demonstrate that the great vessels are arising from the "wrong" ventricle. The aorta runs anterior and to right of the pulmonary artery. Additionally, the great vessels have a parallel course instead of crossing each other (Fig. 6.5). Another feature is an abnormal three-vessel-trachea view in which only the aortic arch on the left side and the superior vena cava on the right side can be identified (Fig. 6.6). The pulmonary artery is positioned inferior to the aorta and thus not visible in the three-vessel view in transposition of the great arteries.

Examination of the great arteries is important to diagnose common arterial trunk. Inclining the transducer cranially will reveal a large, single great vessel that overrides a

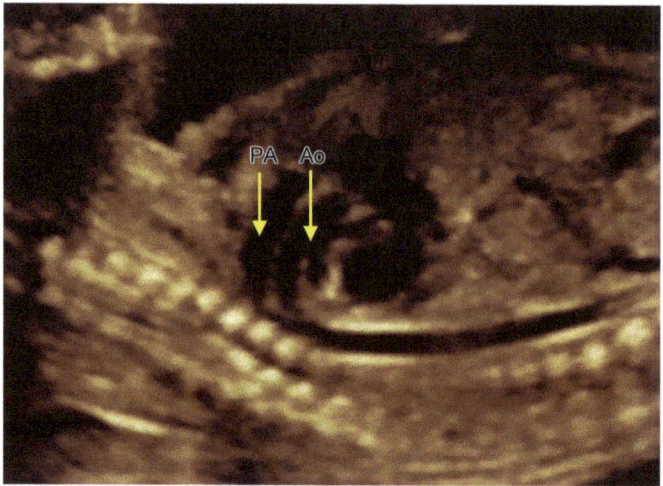

**Fig. 6.5:** Sagittal view in transposition of the great arteries showing the presence of parallel, rather than crossing, great arteries arising form the ventricles. (PA: Pulmonary artery; Ao: Aorta)

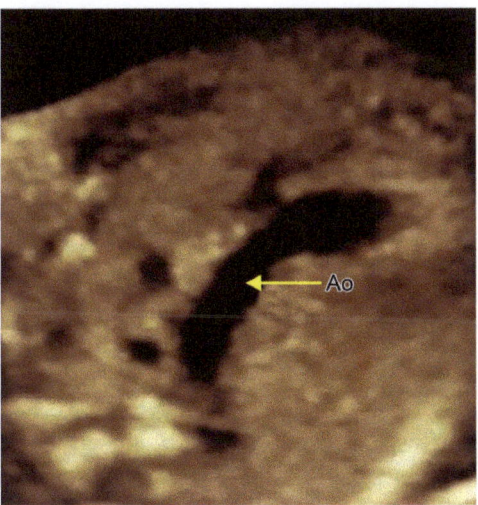

**Fig. 6.6:** Three vessel view in transposition of the great arteries showing the absence of the pulmonary artery as running below and parallel to the aorta. (Ao: Aorta)

ventricular septal defect. Further anterior angulation of the transducer confirms that there is only a single great vessel with branches to the pulmonary, systemic, and coronary circulations arising from the heart (Fig. 6.7). A large, malaligned outlet ventricular septal defect is a common association. Common arterial trunk, pulmonary atresia with ventricular septal defect, and tetralogy of Fallot are difficult to discern from each other on prenatal echocardiography. Visualization of the branch pulmonary arteries off of the common trunk is together with thickened valve leaflets are more in favor of common arterial trunk and less likely in pulmonary atresia with ventricular septal defect and tetralogy of Fallot.

In poor maternal glycemic control-related fetal hyperglycemia, glycogen can accumulate in the cardiac muscle and growth will be stimulated by the hyperinsulinism due to fetal pancreas hyperstimulation. This hypertrophy can obstruct the cardiac blood flow and even cause cardiac failure. Hypertrophic subaortic stenosis has been reported in very severe cases.[25,26] One of the common explanation for the unexplained death in late pregnancy of fetuses of diabetic patients, is this phenomena.[27] However, the absolute prenatal risk of a hypertrophic myocardiopathy in pregnant women with diabetes and the adequate management and interventions are still poorly understood. Additionally, further studies including larger number of cases with accurate postnatal follow-up are warranted to reach a cutoff value of the septal thickness for the prenatal prediction of symptomatic cardiomyopathy in infants of diabetic mothers.

Hypertrophic myocardiopathy is characterized by hypertrophy of the interventricular septum and the ventricular walls. The interventricular septum should be measured in its midway part in the 4-chamber view with the ultrasound beam perpendicular to the interventricular septum preferably in the end-diastolic phase. Hypertrophic myocardiopathy can be suspected if the interventricular septum measures more than 5 mm (Fig. 6.7).

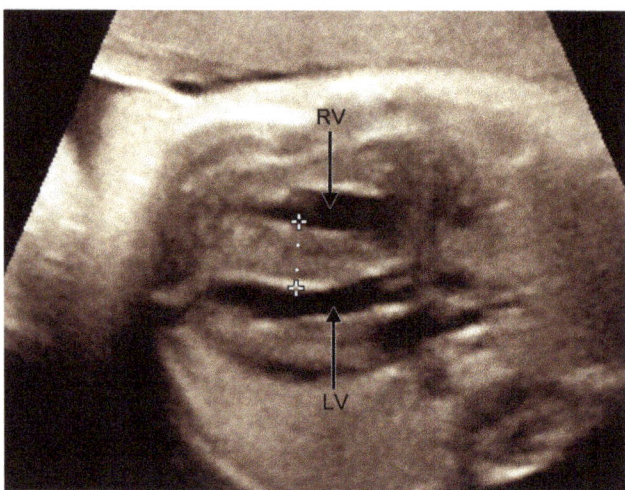

**Fig. 6.7:** Hypertrophic myocardiopathy with hypertrophy of the interventricular septum measuring more than 5 mm. (RV: Right ventricle; LV: Left ventricle)

## CENTRAL NERVOUS SYSTEM ANOMALIES AND NEURAL TUBE DEFECTS

The incidence of neural tube defect in the diabetic obstetric population is increased when compared with the nondiabetic one (approximately 20/1,000 vs 1–2/1,000). Neural tube defects can be roughly subdivided into open and closed types. The open type is further subdivided in two types (1) myelomeningocele and (2) myelocele, which are both distinguished clinically by protrusion of the neural placode through a midline bony and skin defect on the back. Myelomeningoceles account for more than 98% of open spina bifida while myeloceles are rather rare. The main difference between a myelomeningocele and myelocele is the position of the neural placode relative to the spinal canal. The neural placode is outside the spinal canal and protrudes above the skin surface with a myelomeningocele (Fig. 6.8) and is inside the spinal canal and flush with the skin surface with a myelocele (Fig. 6.9).

Improved image resolution in the last 30 years has led to a marked improvement of ultrasound diagnosis of open spina bifida. The vast majority of cases with open spina bifida are now being detected at second trimester screening. However, ultrasound diagnosis can be limited because of a dorso-posterior position of the fetus. Accurate diagnosis of open spina bifida requires a thorough examination of spine and intactness of the overlying skin. However, the later is difficult to demonstrate in myelocele in which there is no cystic structure above the skin defect (Fig. 6.9). The only reliable way to diagnose open spina bifida is thus through a thorough examination of the posterior fossa. Typical abnormal shape of the cerebellum due to its dorso-caudal displacement into the spinal canal (so-called banana sign) with obliteration of the cisterna magna (Chiari II malformation) (Fig. 6.10) is pathognomonic for open spina bifida and will lead to the diagnosis.[28] Recent first trimester ultrasound studies have shown that signs of caudal displacement of the posterior brain stem are present in fetuses with open

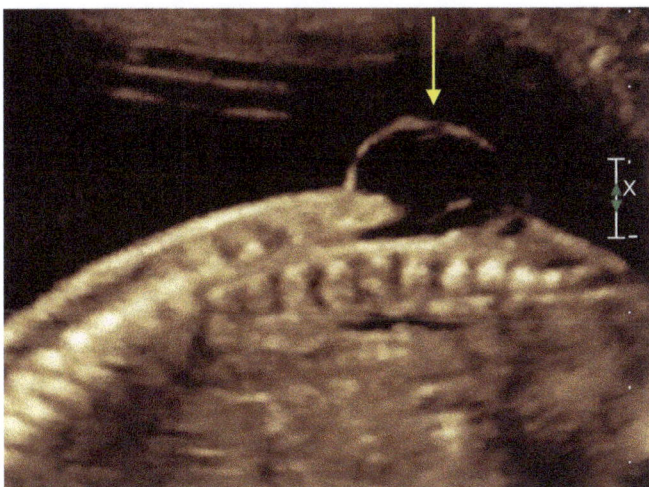

**Fig. 6.8:** Lumbosacral myelomeningoceles with the neural placode protruding above the skin surface (arrow).

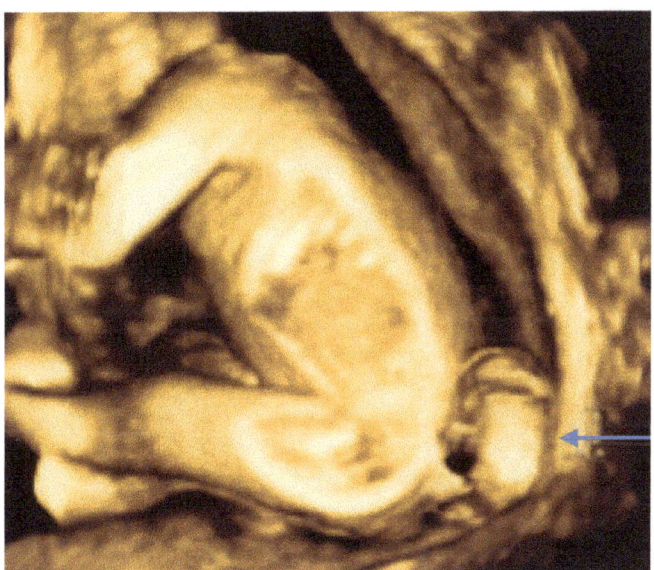

**Fig. 6.9:** 3D-Rendering of a lumbosacral myelomeningocele protruding above the skin.

spina bifida as early as 11–14 weeks' gestation. This displacement causes enlargement of the fourth ventricle by compression of the cisterna magna (Figs. 6.11 and 6.12). As a consequence, the so-called intracranial translucency will be absent.[29]

Anencephaly is with a rate of 1/200 diabetic pregnancies a common complication of diabetic pregnancies. It is easily diagnosed as characterized by absent bony calvarium and prominent bulging eyes. Microcephaly is another CNS malformation associated with diabetes in pregnancy.

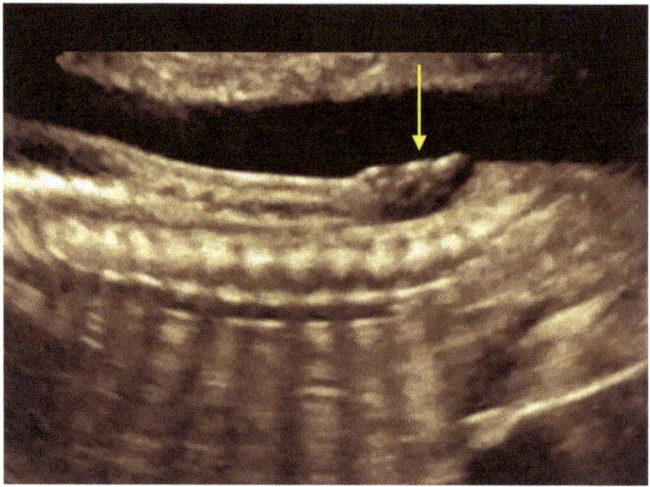

**Fig. 6.10:** Myelocele with the neural placode flush with the skin surface.

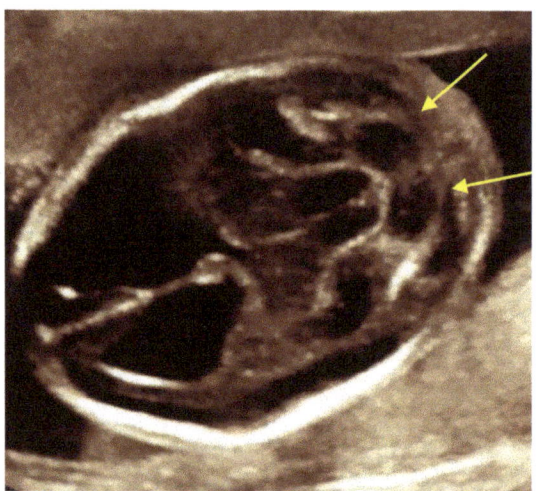

**Fig. 6.11:** Posterior fossa in open spina bifida. Not the absence of the cisterna magna and the abnormal shape of the cerebellum (so called banana sign).

## GASTROINTESTINAL ANOMALIES

Imperforate anus is one of the most common gastrointestinal malformations associated with diabetes. An imperforate anus had been thought to be difficult to diagnose prenatally. However, prenatal diagnosis by direct visualization of the fetal perineum has been reported.[30-33] The fetal anal structures are best visualized on tangential views of the fetal perineum. The normal fetal anus appears as hypoechogenic ring surrounding the hyperechogenic anal mucosa (so-called "target" sign) (Fig. 6.13). Characteristic images of anal atresia are the nonvisualization of

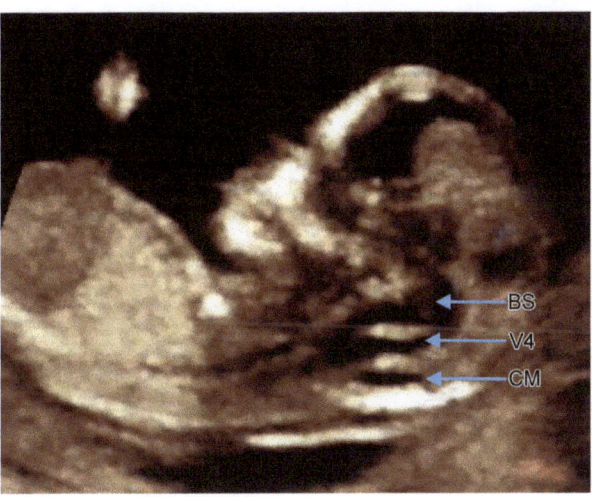

**Fig. 6.12:** Normal mid-sagittal plane of the fetal brain in the first trimester showing brainstem (BS), fourth ventricle (V4) and cisterna magna (CM).

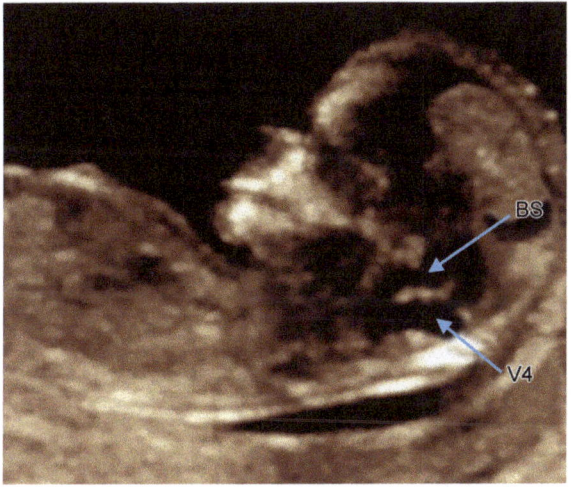

**Fig. 6.13:** Abnormal mid-sagittal plane of the fetal brain in the first trimester. The fourth ventricle (V4) appears enlarged and the cisterna magna is not visible (BS: Brainstem; V4: Fourth ventricle).

the anal sphincter muscles and anal mucosa and only a hyperechoic linear line across the perineum (Fig. 6.14). Prenatal assessment of the anal sphincter can help in the diagnosis of anorectal atresia in a high-risk population including the diabetic one (Fig. 6.15).[32] Again, imperforate anus is considered by some authors as a variation of the caudal regression.

## FEMORAL HYPOPLASIA-UNUSUAL FACIES SYNDROME

The association of the so-called femoral hypoplasia-unusual facies syndrome with maternal insulin-dependent diabetes is well recognized.[34,35] Patients suffering from the femoral

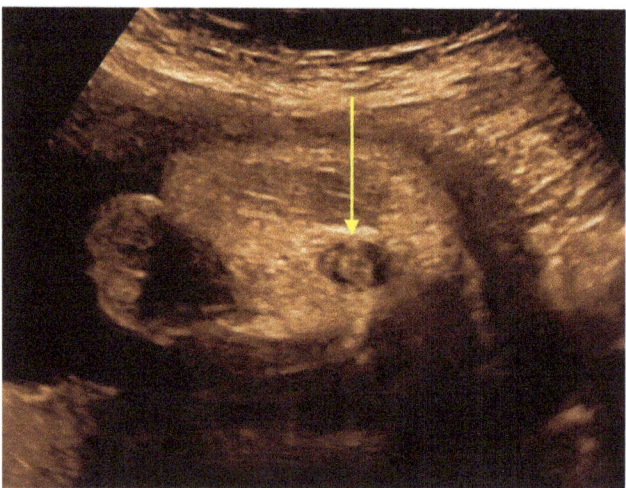

**Fig. 6.14:** Normal anal sphincter muscles appears as hypoechogenic ring surrounding the hyperechogenic anal mucosa (so called "target" sign).

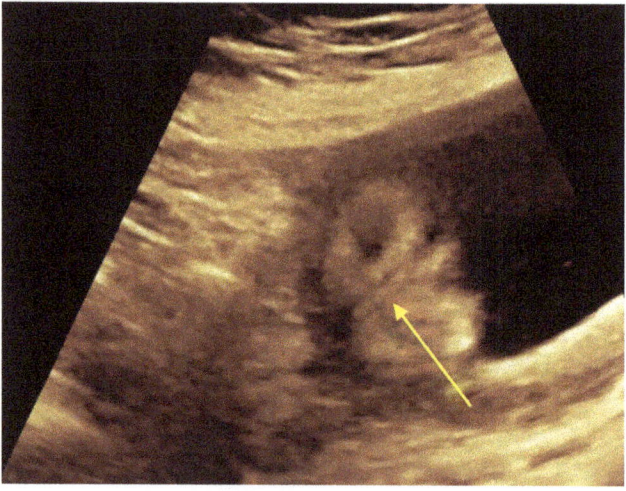

**Fig. 6.15:** Nonvisualization of the anal sphincter muscles and anal mucosa and only a hyperechoic linear line across the perineum in anal atresia (arrow).

hypoplasia-unusual facies syndrome are characterized by a variable degree of unilateral or bilateral femoral hypoplasia associated with facial clefting and occasionally other minor anomalies. Affected fetuses have a broad spectrum of associated malformations that occur with variable frequency including malformations involving the upper limbs, ribs, vertebrae or central nervous system, such as neuronal migrational disorders and agenesis of the corpus callosum. Assessment of the femoral length and appearance in the fetus diabetic mothers is of critical importance as these parameters could represent as markers of multiple malformations.

## IDEAL WINDOW TO PERFORM THE "SCREENING" ULTRASOUND EXAMINATION

Using the transvaginal approach it is easier to visualize fetal anatomical structures in early pregnancy. However, a thorough fetal evaluation cannot be completed only after a second trimester routine anatomical scan. In particular, the central nervous system is constantly developing throughout pregnancy. The corpus callosum as well as the gyri and the sulci develop slowly and anomalies cannot be ruled out until before 22 weeks' gestation. In the same line, it has been shown that interrogation of the fetal heart is already feasible at the end of the first trimester. However, at 22 weeks' gestation, the heart is larger, which allows clearer views for precise diagnosis. Thus, an early scan at 10–14 weeks of gestation will allow the exclusion of major malformations while an additional scan at 20–22 weeks remains important in order to rule out possible previously missed malformations. One should bear in mind that ultrasound examination of obese diabetic pregnancies showed up to suboptimal image quality in up to 37% of the cases and incomplete examinations with repeat examinations in up to 17% of the cases. The malformation detection rate was markedly reduced in diabetic women when compared with the low-risk population (30% vs 73%).[36]

## REFERENCES

1. Kitzmiller JL, Buchanan TA, Kjos S, et al. Pre-conception care of diabetes, congenital malformations, and spontaneous abortions. Diabetes Care. 1996;19(5):514-41.
2. Sheffield JS, Butler-Koster EL, Casey BM, et al. Maternal diabetes mellitus and infant malformations. Obstet Gynecol. 2002;100(5 Pt 1):925-30.
3. Sharpe PB, Chan A, Haan EA, et al. Maternal diabetes and congenital anomalies in South Australia 1986-2000: a population-based cohort study. Birth Defects Res A Clin Mol Teratol. 2005;73(9):605-11.
4. Lapolla A, Dalfrà MG, Bonomo M, et al. Gestational diabetes mellitus in Italy: a multicenter study. Eur J Obstet Gynecol Reprod Biol. 2009;145(2):149-53.
5. Hod M, Rabinerson D, Kaplan B, et al. Perinatal complications following gestational diabetes mellitus how 'sweet' is ill? Acta Obstet Gynecol Scand. 1996;75(9):809-15.
6. Lisowski LA, Verheijen PM, Copel JA, et al. Congenital heart disease in pregnancies complicated by maternal diabetes mellitus. An international clinical collaboration, literature review, and meta-analysis. Herz. 2010;35(1):19-26.
7. Shaw GM, Quach T, Nelson V, et al. Neural tube defects associated with maternal periconceptional dietary intake of simple sugars and glycemic index. Am J Clin Nutr. 2003;78(5):972-8.
8. Yazdy MM, Mitchell AA, Liu S, et al. Maternal dietary glycaemic intake during pregnancy and the risk of birth defects. Paediatr Perinat Epidemiol. 2011;25(4):340-6.
9. Hawthorne G, Robson S, Ryall EA, et al. Prospective population based survey of outcome of pregnancy in diabetic women: results of the Northern Diabetic Pregnancy Audit, 1994. BMJ. 1997;315(7103):279-81.
10. Duhamel B. From the mermaid to anal imperforation: the syndrome of caudal regression. Arch Dis Child. 1961;36(186):152-55.
11. Kucera J. Rate and type of congenital anomalies among offspring of diabetic women. J Reprod Med. 1971;7(2):73-82.
12. Mills JL. Malformations in infants of diabetic mothers. Teratology. 1982;25(3):385-94.
13. Al Kaissi A, Klaushofer K, Grill F. Caudal regression syndrome and popliteal webbing in connection with maternal diabetes mellitus: a case report and literature review. Cases J. 2008;1(1):407.

14. Gabbe SG. Congenital malformations in infants of diabetic mothers. Obstet Gynecol Surv. 1977;32(3):125-32.
15. Pedersen J, Molsted-Pedersen LM. Congenital malformations: the possible role of diabetes care outside pregnancy. Ciba Found Symp. 1978;(63):265-71.
16. Fuhrmann K, Reiher H, Semmler K, et al. Prevention of congenital malformations in infants of insulin-dependent diabetic mothers. Diabetes Care. 1983;6(3):219-23.
17. Kitzmiller JL, Younger MD, Hare JW, et al. Continuous subcutaneous insulin therapy during early pregnancy. Obstet Gynecol. 1985;66(5):606-11.
18. Lowy C, Beard RW, Goldschmidt J. Congenital malformations in babies of diabetic mothers. Diabet Med. 1986;3(5):458-62.
19. Becerra JE, Khoury MJ, Cordero JF, et al. Diabetes mellitus during pregnancy and the risks for specific birth defects: a population-based case-control study. Pediatrics. 1990;85(1):1-9.
20. Meyer BA, Palmer SM. Pregestational diabetes. Semin Perinatol. 1990;14(1):12-23.
21. Rosenn B, Miodovnik M, Combs CA, et al. Glycemic thresholds for spontaneous abortion and congenital malformations in insulin-dependent diabetes mellitus. Obstet Gynecol. 1994;84(4):515-20.
22. Agha MM, Glazier RH, Moineddin R, et al. Congenital abnormalities in newborns of women with pregestational diabetes: a time-trend analysis, 1994 to 2009. Birth Defects Res A Clin Mol Teratol. 2016;106(10):831-9.
23. Landon MB, Gabbe SG, Diabetes and pregnancy. Med Clin North Am. 1988;72(6):1493-511.
24. Shields LE, Gan EA, Murphy HF, et al. The prognostic value of hemoglobin A1c in predicting fetal heart disease in diabetic pregnancies. Obstet Gynecol. 1993;81(6):954-7.
25. Veille JC, Hanson R, Sivakoff M, et al. Fetal cardiac size in normal, intrauterine growth retarded, and diabetic pregnancies. Am J Perinatol. 1993;10(4):275-9.
26. Kozák-Bárány A, Jokinen E, Kero P, et al. Impaired left ventricular diastolic function in newborn infants of mothers with pregestational or gestational diabetes with good glycemic control. Early Hum Dev. 2004;77(1-2):13-22.
27. Rizzo G, Arduini D, Romanini C. Accelerated cardiac growth and abnormal cardiac flow in fetuses of type I diabetic mothers. Obstet Gynecol. 1992;80(3 Pt 1):369-76.
28. Bahlmann F, Reinhard I, Schramm T, et al. Cranial and cerebral signs in the diagnosis of spina bifida between 18 and 22 weeks of gestation: a German multicentre study. Prenat Diagn. 2015;35(3):228-35.
29. Chaoui R, Benoit B, Mitkowska-Wozniak H, et al. Assessment of intracranial translucency (IT) in the detection of spina bifida at the 11-13-week scan. Ultrasound Obstet Gynecol. 2009;34(3):249-52.
30. Elchalal U, Yanai N, Valsky DV, et al. Application of 3-dimensional ultrasonography to imaging the fetal anal canal. J Ultrasound Med. 2010;29(8):1195-201.
31. Vijayaraghavan SB, Prema AS, Suganyadevi P. Sonographic depiction of the fetal anus and its utility in the diagnosis of anorectal malformations. J Ultrasound Med. 2011;30(1):37-45.
32. Ochoa JH, Chiesa M, Vildoza RP, et al. Evaluation of the perianal muscular complex in the prenatal diagnosis of anorectal atresia in a high-risk population. Ultrasound Obstet Gynecol. 2012;39(5):521-7.
33. Lee MY, Won HS, Shim JY, et al. Sonographic determination of type in a fetal imperforate anus. J Ultrasound Med. 2016;35(6):1285-91.
34. Daentl DL, Smith DW, Scott Cl, et al. Femoral hypoplasia-unusual facies syndrome. J Pediatr. 1975;86(1):107-11.
35. Paladini D, Maruotti GM, Sglavo G, et al. Diagnosis of femoral hypoplasia-unusual facies syndrome in the fetus. Ultrasound Obstet Gynecol. 2007;30(3):354-8.
36. Wong SF, Chan FY, Cincotta RB, et al. Routine ultrasound screening in diabetic pregnancies. Ultrasound Obstet Gynecol. 2002;19(2):171-6.

# Chapter 7

# Offspring of Diabetic Mother

*Milan Stanojevic*

## INTRODUCTION

A positive family history, older maternal age, and increased obesity were well established as the risk factors for development of gestational diabetes mellitus (GDM) in the last more than 60 years, while changing the lifestyle has contributed to increase in GDM prevalence from 3.1% to 8.5% in different ethnic groups, which is shown in the Figure 7.1.[1] In Japan, for instance, the incidence of GDM has increased by 4.1-fold from 2.9% to 12.1% in the 20-year period.[2] A mother who gave birth to macrosomic infants with birth weight over 4,000 g is at higher risk of development of gestational diabetes in the subsequent pregnancy.[3] Worldwide number of women of reproductive age with diabetes mellitus is currently about 60 million, and this number will double by 2030.[4]

Although the underlying pathophysiology of type 1 and GDM/type 2 diabetes is different, the effects on the mothers and fetuses are the same—maternal and fetal hyperglycemia, regardless of the fact that the metabolic milieu for the fetus is different when there is primarily disorder of insulin resistance (type 1 diabetes) or beta-cell dysfunction (type 2 diabetes/GDM).[5]

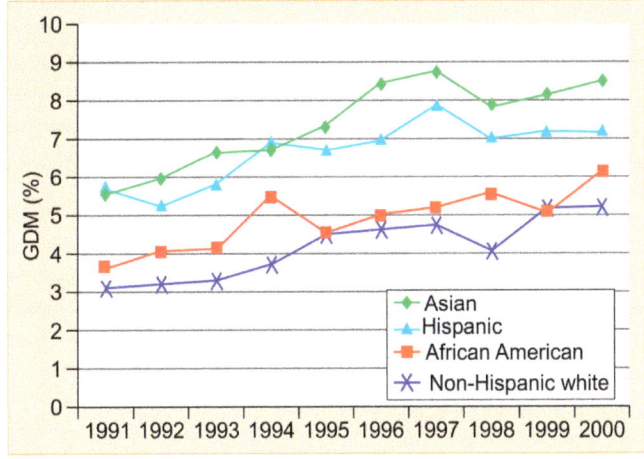

**Fig. 7.1:** Age-adjusted prevalence of gestational diabetes mellitus (GDM) by race/ethnicity and years: Northern California Kaiser Permanente, 1991–2000.[1]

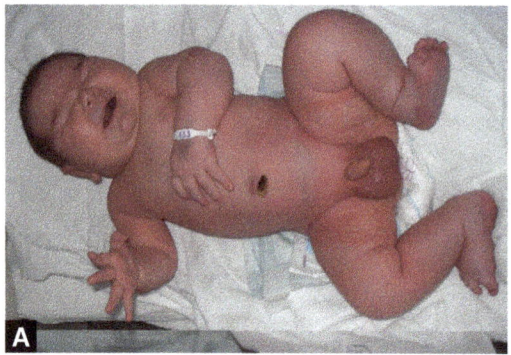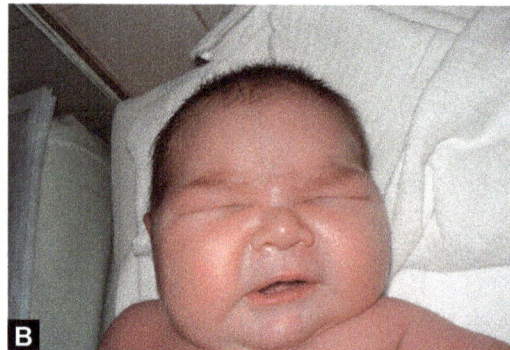

**Figs. 7.2A and B:** Typical appearance of the newborn infant from poorly regulated diabetic pregnancy.

Pedersen was the one who almost 70 years ago proved the effect of maternal hyperglycemia on the fetus, producing fetal hyperinsulinemia providing to the most of the fetal and neonatal consequences like deposition of large amounts of body fat giving the infant its characteristic appearance (Figs. 7.2A and B), with increased body weight and hypertrophic growth compared with subjects from nondiabetic pregnancies.[6] Maternal diabetes may be pregestational (type 1 or type 2 diabetes diagnosed before pregnancy with a prevalence rate of about 1.8%) or diabetes diagnosed during pregnancy (GDM) with a prevalence rate of 7.5%.[7,8]

In low- and middle-income countries (LMIC), consumption of refined carbohydrates, sugars and fats is increased resulting with the increased prevalence of diabetes, obesity, overweight, cardiovascular, and other noncommunicable diseases.[8] The increased prevalence of GDM in high-income countries (the United Kingdom from 2% to 3%, and in the United States of America from 2% to 10%) is caused by the same reasons as in the LMIC (prevalence in south of India 13.9%, in Brazil 7.6%, and 109% prevalence increase in Africa),[8] which undoubtedly represents a serious public health burden.[3] Introduction of the modern lifestyles in LMIC is obviously responsible for the epidemic of obesity and older maternal age, which both may contribute to an increased prevalence of GDM.[1] GDM is associated with increased prevalence of perinatal complications in the mother and her offspring and they both have increased the risk of developing obesity, diabetes, or so-called metabolic syndrome later in life.[1] The assessment of the trends in GDM prevalence is important for development of appropriate strategies to prevent postpartum diabetes.[1]

The more general aspect of disturbed intrauterine growth raised by David Barker and colleagues in 1980s known as Barker hypothesis, nowadays known as Developmental Origins of Health and Disease (DOHaD), stated that major causes of cardiovascular and metabolic diseases in adulthood originate from impaired intrauterine development.[9,10] Pregestational diabetes increases the risk of an impaired intrauterine environment as well as unrecognized or poorly controlled GDM.[9,10] Early fetal and neonatal complications of maternal diabetes are well understood, while molecular mechanisms of long-term offspring consequences due to hyperglycemia are not.[11-13] In order to maintain the health of diabetic mothers and their infants in the short- and the long-term, it is important to maintain the glycemic control before and during pregnancy to improve the health of the next generation.[2]

## FETAL EFFECTS OF MATERNAL HYPERGLYCEMIA

Maternal hyperglycemia may affect the fetus adversely throughout the whole pregnancy—spontaneous abortion and major birth defects in the first trimester, and in the second, and the third trimesters fetal hyperglycemia, hyperinsulinemia, and macrosomia.[3] Higher oxygen consumption rates and relative fetal hypoxemia due to fetal hyperinsulinemia may result in alterations in fetal iron distribution and erythropoiesis, metabolic acidosis, and increased fetal mortality.[3] Insulin-sensitive tissues like liver, muscle, cardiac muscle, and subcutaneous fat are insulin sensitive and contribute to fetal macrosomia, and defined as body weight above the 90th percentile for gestational age.[3] Besides that fetal hyperinsulinemia contributes to the delayed lung maturation, increased synthesis of erythropoietin leading to polycythemia, increased catecholamine production providing to the development of hypertrophic cardiomyopathy, and altered neurodevelopment.[3] The risk of stillbirth in poorly controlled diabetic pregnancies is as high as 20–30%.[14]

## NEONATAL EFFECTS OF MATERNAL HYPERGLYCEMIA

Maternal hyperglycemia may lead to the following neonatal complications—macrosomia, prematurity, respiratory distress syndrome, perinatal asphyxia, hypoglycemia and hypocalcemia, polycythemia and hyperviscosity, hyperbilirubinemia, low-iron stores, congenital anomalies, and cardiomyopathy.[15] The following relative frequencies of complications were found in the study of 530 infants born to the mothers with GDM and 177 mothers with insulin-dependent diabetes mellitus (IDDM) from 1994 to 1996:[15]

- Almost ten times increased a risk of perinatal mortality
- Percentage of newborns admitted to neonatal intensive care was 47%
- Prematurity rate was around 36%
- Large for the gestational age (LGA) defined as the birth weight above the 90th percentile for gestational age observed in 36%
- Respiratory distress found in 34%
- Hyperbilirubinemia diagnosed in 25%
- Polycythemia found in 5%
- Congenital anomalies observed in 5%
- Small for gestational age diagnosed in 2%.

Similar data were found in the recent study, without a difference in birth trauma rate between the newborns from nondiabetic and diabetic pregnancies.[16] Diabetic mothers with better-controlled glycemia during pregnancy in terms of lower glycated albumin and glycated hemoglobin levels gave birth to the newborns who had a lower incidence of hyperglycemia, which is the main source of all neonatal complications, as Pedersen stated many decades ago.[17] Glycated albumin, which is independent of iron deficiency during pregnancy, showed to be the better indicator of adverse neonatal outcome (hypoglycemia, respiratory disorders, hypocalcemia, myocardial hypertrophy, and large-for-dates status) than glycated hemoglobin.[2,17]

## PERINATAL OUTCOME OF THE OFFSPRING FROM DIABETIC PREGNANCIES

Perinatal outcome in diabetic pregnancies is dependent on the diagnostic criteria applied in diabetic pregnancies are influencing perinatal outcome and the assessment of perinatal risk.[17,18] Recently, the United Kingdom's National Institute for Health and Care Excellence (NICE) recommended new diagnostic thresholds for GDM, which are different from the International Association of the Diabetes and Pregnancy Study Groups (IADPSG) criteria endorsed by the World Health Organization (WHO).[18] The IADPSG criteria identify women at substantial risk of complications who would not be identified by the NICE 2015 criteria.[18]

In the study of 18,005 newborns, 996 were macrosomic infants (5.53%), among whom 103 (10.3%) were born to diabetic mothers.[16] Diabetic mothers had higher parity (1.89 vs. 1.35; $P < 0.000$), cesarean section rate (52.4 vs. 31.1%; $P < 0.05$), neonatal resuscitation rate (5.8 vs. 1.8%; $P < 0.006$; relative risk—RR: 2.9; 95% confidence interval—CI: 1.42–5.9), and greater need for neonatal hospitalization (19.4 vs. 9.6%; $P < 0.002$; RR: 2; 95% CI: 1.3–3.2) and intensive care (5.8 vs. 0.7%; $P < 0.000$; RR: 5.3; 95% CI: 2.8–10) mostly for hypoglycemia (7.8 vs. 1%; $P < 0.000$; RR: 5; 95% CI: 2.8–8.3), jaundice (8.7 vs. 2.1%; $P < 0.000$; RR: 3.1; 95% CI: 1.9–5.9), respiratory distress (4.9 vs. 1.3%; $P < 0.009$; RR: 2.9; 95% CI: 1.4–6.7), and asphyxia (2.9 vs. 0.4%; $P < 0.005$; RR: 4.3; 95% CI: 1.8–11.1).[16] No differences were found in birth trauma.[16]

In another study of 10,781 extremely preterm infants, 536 (5%) were born to women with IDDM of whom 58% had insulin therapy before pregnancy, and 36% had insulin therapy during pregnancy.[19] Infants of mothers with insulin therapy before pregnancy had higher risks of necrotizing enterocolitis [adjusted RR = 1.55 (95% CI 1.17–2.05)] and late-onset sepsis [adjusted RR = 1.26 (95% CI 1.07–1.48)] than infants of mothers without IDDM.[19] There was some indication of higher inhospital mortality risk among infants of mothers with insulin therapy before pregnancy compared with those of the mothers with insulin therapy during pregnancy [adjusted RR = 1.33 (95% CI 1.00–1.79)].[19] Among survivors evaluated at 18–22 months corrected age, average head circumference Z score was lower for infants of the mothers with insulin therapy before pregnancy, compared with those without IDDM, but there were no differences in the risk of neurodevelopmental impairment.[19]

The data from the recently published study on the risk of development of the retinopathy of prematurity (ROP) and stage 1 ROP showed that the presence of maternal diabetes is significantly associated with the development of ROP and stage 1 ROP in premature infants with a birth weight of 1,500 g or more.[20]

## INHOSPITAL CARE FOR THE NEWBORNS FROM DIABETIC PREGNANCIES

It is well known that newborns from diabetic pregnancies have a higher risk of hospitalization and treatment in the neonatal intensive care than newborns from nondiabetic pregnancies.[15-17] In published studies, the data are quite variable due to different treatment criteria. In one study, there were 47% of newborns from diabetic pregnancies who needed neonatal intensive care.[15] According to the study by Lloreda-García and ass. macrosomic newborns from diabetic pregnancies had been more often hospitalized (19.4 vs. 9.6%; P <0.002; RR: 2; 95% CI: 1.3–3.2), with increased rates of admissions to the neonatal intensive care (5.8 vs. 0.7%; P <0.000; RR: 5.3; 95% CI: 2.8–10).[16]

In the paper from Saudi Arabia, a total of 601 infants were enrolled in the study consisting of 319 infants of nondiabetic mothers, and 282 infants of diabetic mothers, showing that infants of diabetic mothers had significantly higher rates of associated complications, causing increased admission rate to the neonatal intensive care unit (NICU) when compared with infants of nondiabetic mothers.[21] There was no difference in the rate of complications between infants of mothers who had gestational diabetics and those with pregestational diabetes.[21]

Complications in the offspring from diabetic pregnancy, regardless of the cause of the disorder, arise due to their exposure to intrauterine conditions adversely affecting placental and fetal development.[22,23] Such adverse conditions in diabetic pregnancies have been associated with alterations in anatomy and physiology of the placenta, mainly based on changes on the microanatomical and/or even molecular level, including aberrant villous vascularization, a disbalance of vasoactive molecules, and enhanced oxidative stress.[22,23] In experimental rat model and in the research on human placentas, it has been proved that impaired fetal oxygenation and changes in transplacental nutrient supply were the main causes of the metabolic syndrome in the offspring.[22,23] Although transplacental glucose flux is flow limited and independent of glucose transporter availability, transport of essential and nonessential amino acids and expression of genes involved in lipid transport and metabolism are significantly affected by GDM in humans and in the animal models.[23]

## RESPIRATORY PATHOLOGY IN NEONATES FROM DIABETIC PREGNANCIES

Respiratory distress syndrome or transient tachypnea of the newborn is the result of delayed fetal pulmonary maturation of the infants of diabetic mothers, but the risk of fetal death, fetal overgrowth, and neonatal birth trauma is also considerably increased.[24] It has been proven in current studies concerning the good maternal metabolic control of the mothers with preexisting gestational diabetes or GDM complicated with impaired glucose homeostasis is insufficient to ensure normal oxygenation and appropriate metabolic milieu for the fetus.[25] In the gestational diabetes rat experimental model, authors proved that the rat fetuses of the diabetic group presented a delay in lung histogenesis and in the differentiation of the type II pneumocytes, accompanied by a decreased level of protein D associated to surfactant.[26] This was probably one of the reasons, why respiratory disorders were diagnosed in 48.4% of infants of diabetic mothers and only in 12.6% of newborns of healthy mothers (P <0.01), with 42% of infants of diabetic mothers and 19.7% of infants of healthy mothers who needed additional oxygen treatment.[27] In macrosomic newborns born to diabetic mothers, the incidence of respiratory distress was 4.2% compared with only 1.3% incidence of respiratory distress in macrosomic infants from nondiabetic mothers with a RR of 2.9 with 95% CI between 1.4 and 6.7; P < 0.009.[16]

The risk of the adverse perinatal outcome in offspring of mothers with type 1 diabetes and GDM did not differ by sex, except for a higher risk in male infants for respiratory disorders.[28]

The current paradigm of delaying delivery to 39 weeks in women with controlled and uncomplicated diabetes has been challenged by recent evidence advocating delivery by 38 weeks to improve perinatal outcomes by decreasing the risk of stillbirth.[24] Additional well-designed and adequately powered prospective studies are needed to better understand the short- and long-term implications of the optimal timing of delivery in this high-risk population.[24] Use of the automated lamellar body count in amniotic fluid could be a good method for detection of lung maturity before delivery, which has been proposed by some authors as a promising method.[29]

## HYPERTROPHIC CARDIOMYOPATHY AND OFFSPRING OF DIABETIC MOTHER

As already pointed out several times, hypoglycemia is the most common transient and potentially serious consequence of hyperinsulinism arising in the asphyxiated, small for gestational age infants, and infants of a diabetic mothers.[16,24] Sometimes, it should be differentiated with hypoglycemia caused by congenital hyperinsulinism, which is the most common cause of hypoglycemia in children.[30] In the past 20 years, it has become apparent that hyperinsulinism is caused by genetic defects in the pathways that regulate pancreatic beta-cell insulin secretion.[30] Eleven genes are associated with monogenic forms of hyperinsulinism—*ABCC8, KCNJ11, GLUD1, GCK, HADH1, UCP2, MCT1, HNF4A, HNF1A, HK1, PGM1*, while syndromic hyperinsulinism may be a part of Beckwith-Wiedemann, Kabuki, Turner, and other syndromes.[30]

Hyperinsulinism, among other, may cause cardiac problems in newborns.[31] The mechanisms by which insulin causes cardiac problems have not been defined, but the heart is an important insulin target, and expression of functional insulin receptors by the cardiomyocyte is comparable with that of other insulin-sensitive cells.[31] Downstream of the insulin receptor, glycogen synthase kinase-3-beta negatively regulates cardiac hypertrophy.[31] Expression of enzyme glycogen synthase kinase-3-beta is inhibited by insulin, which means that it is a potential mechanism for hypertrophic cardiomyopathy in the hyperinsulinemic fetuses.[31] In infants of diabetic mothers, besides hypertrophic cardiomyopathy, the following echocardiographic findings have been found—in 70% patent ductus arteriosus, in 68% patent foramen ovale, in 5% atrial septal defect, in 4% small muscular ventricular septal defect, in 2% mitral valve prolapse, and in 1% pulmonary stenosis.[32] Severe forms of congenital heart defects like D-transposition of great arteries, tetralogy of Fallot, and hypoplastic left heart syndrome (1% each) were found in the group of infants of diabetic mothers, while isolated aortic stenosis and coarctation of aorta were not encountered in this series.[32] The overall incidence of congenital heart defects was 15% excluding patent ductus arteriosus and patent foramen ovale and hypertrophic cardiomyopathy.[32] Hypertrophic cardiomyopathy mainly expressed as the hypertrophic interventricular septum in that study was observed in 38% of cases.[32]

It is questionable, how often hypertrophic cardiomyopathy can be diagnosed in newborns with hyperinsulinism.[31,32] In the study of infants with congenital hyperinsulinism, hypertrophic cardiomyopathy was identified in 15% (95% CI 6–23%), resolving in all of them after treatment.[31] In newborns of diabetic mothers, hypertrophic cardiomyopathy may remain unrecognized. The incidence of cardiomyopathy in infants of diabetic mothers is difficult to determine, as few studies have prospectively performed echocardiograms in infants of diabetic mothers.[31] In the recent study of 35 infants of diabetic mothers compared with 35 infants from the control group, the interventricular septum thickness in case group was higher as compared with the control group (at end systole = 6.61 ± 1.64 mm vs. 5.75 ± 0.95 mm, P = 0.0371; at end-diastole = 4.61 ± 1.59 mm vs. 3.42 ± 0.70 mm, P = 0.0001).[33] A risk ratio of 2.333 (CI 0.656–8.298) was obtained for ventricular septum hypertrophy, with a higher risk for the newborns of the mothers with gestational than pregestational diabetes.[33] Besides conventional echocardiography, there is a possibility to use more sophisticated methods of echocardiographic investigation like tissue Doppler imaging (TDI) and two-dimensional speckle-tracking imaging (STI) like in the study of 45 infants of diabetic mothers and the same number of control infants.[34] It has been shown that even when conventional echocardiography showed normal findings, TDI, and STI found to be sensitive tools able to early detect cardiac dysfunction in infants of diabetic mothers, which have not been correlated with maternal or fetal HBA1c findings.[34]

Diazoxide, an adenosine triphosphate-sensitive potassium ($K_{ATP}$) channel agonist, has been the primary drug for infants with hyperinsulinism for the last 50 years.[30] In the majority of infants with monogenic hyperinsulinism and mutations of *ABCC8* or *KCNJ11*, diazoxide is ineffective.[30] In the study including case reports and case series, a total number of 619 patients treated for congenital hyperinsulinism, drugs used were diazoxide (in 84% of patients), somatostatin analogs (16%), calcium channel antagonists (4%), and glucagon (1%).[35] The mean duration of diazoxide treatment until remission was 57 months, while mean duration of treatment with somatostatin analogs until remission was 49 months.[35] Infants with hypertrophic cardiomyopathy due to hyperinsulinism were treated with corticosteroids, which might have played a role in development of hypertrophic cardiomyopathy.[30] Prognosis of infants with hypertrophic cardiomyopathy associated with maternal diabetes is good, while lack of maternal diabetes in pregnancy was connected with a bad prognosis of fetuses with hypertrophic cardiomyopathy.[36]

## OFFSPRING OF DIABETIC MOTHER: PRENATAL AND POSTNATAL GROWTH

Gestational diabetes mellitus and maternal obesity influence the maternal and offspring's health.[12] The global shift toward more Westernized diets resulted in increased consumption of fats, sugars, and refined carbohydrates providing to the increased prevalence of overweight and obesity, diabetes, cardiovascular, and other noncommunicable diseases.[5] Obesity and diabetes in pregnancy have independent and additive effects on maternal and fetal complications.[12]

In a recent meta-analysis including data from 35 papers and over 24,000 infants, offspring (particularly boys) of diabetic mothers (particularly those with gestational diabetes) have greater fat mass than infants of nondiabetic mothers.[37]

It has been shown in another study that maternal prepregnancy body mass index (BMI) and gestational weight gain in the early, mid, and late pregnancy were positively and independently associated with neonatal adiposity.[38] Associations of early- and mid-pregnancy maternal weight gain with neonatal adiposity support the hypothesis that greater maternal weight gain during pregnancy, regardless of prepregnancy BMI, and are directly related to offspring's adiposity at birth.[38] It has been shown in the study relating to shoulder dystocia that women with GDM compared to nondiabetic women had significantly higher prepregnancy body weight, higher prepregnancy BMI, and lower gestational weight gain.[39]

The study of women, infant feeding, and type 2 diabetes after GDM pregnancy, and growth of their offspring (SWIFT offspring study) significantly increased current knowledge about the effects of postnatal feeding on growth during infancy among GDM offspring. This study also lays the foundation for future studies to evaluate the impact of breastfeeding on the GDM offspring's long-term risk of obesity and diabetes.[40] Although the fetus is genetically unique, epigenetic factors like prenatal exposure to impaired maternal glucose metabolism and postnatal newborn feeding practices may influence a growth and disease risk of the offspring in utero and postnatally.[13] It is well known that offspring of diabetic mothers exposed to the impaired metabolic intrauterine environment have an increased risk for overweight and obesity, glucose intolerance, metabolic syndrome, or type 2 diabetes postnatally.[13] Macrosomia of the neonate not connected with GDM and defined as birth weight over 4,000 g is connected with more postnatal complications compared to nonmacrosomic newborns. In the study of 2,766 nondiabetic macrosomic infants, matched to 2,766 control nonmacrosomic infants, the macrosomic group had higher rates of hypoglycemia (1.2% vs. 0.5%, $P = 0.008$), transient tachypnea of the newborn (1.5% vs. 0.5%, $P < 0.001$), hyperthermia (0.6% vs. 0.1%, $P = 0.012$), and birth trauma (2% vs. 0.7%, $P < 0.001$), with no cases of symptomatic polycythemia, and only one case of symptomatic hypoglycemia.[41] Hypoglycemia was positively associated with birth weight, and it was significantly higher in the asymmetric than the symmetric macrosomic newborns.[41] In the study of macrosomic infants from pregnancies without and with GDM, it has been proved that macrosomic infants born to diabetic mothers have an increased risk of hospital admission in the neonatal period for hypoglycemia, jaundice, respiratory distress, and asphyxia, and a greater need of intensive care, while birth trauma rates were similar in both groups.[16]

Obviously, postnatal feeding method of normal newborns (breastfeeding vs. formula feeding) has an influence on postnatal growth as well, which resulted in the publication of new WHO growth standard curves for breastfed infants.[42] Breastfed infants grow more slowly than formula-fed infants, show a greater decline in weight-for-length Z-score between 3 months and 12 months, and tend to be leaner by 12 months to 18 months.[43,44] Breastfeeding may have long-term effects on the growth of the neonates of diabetic mothers, but the evidence is limited to mostly retrospective studies, without taking into account intrauterine metabolic environment and postnatal risk factors, which may influence infant growth.[16] This difference in growth of breastfed and formula-fed infants is probably caused by different protein intake of those two groups of infants with higher protein intake in formula-fed infants. This higher protein intake can produce higher insulin secretion, which has been associated with higher infant BMI later in life.[45] From 5 months of age, the percentage of body fat tends to decline among breastfed infants, while opposite tendency is observed in formula-fed infants.[43,44] This slow down of the postnatal growth of breastfed neonates from pregnancies complicated with GDM is called catch-down growth pattern.[46] Although macrosomic newborns of GDM mothers, compared to macrosomic newborns from nondiabetic pregnancies, are adipose through the 1st year of life, they grow more slowly through the first 2 years of life, with rapid weight gain thereafter providing to the obesity.[47-49] This early postnatal so-called catch-down growth pattern is strongly influenced by a drive to compensate for the intrauterine effects on the fetus of the maternal metabolism associated with obesity and glucose intolerance.[40]

Promotion of breastfeeding is important in general, and particularly in obese and mothers with GDM, because of increased risk of obesity, metabolic syndrome, type 2 diabetes, and many other noncommunicable diseases in their children, which can be decreased by increasing the rate of exclusive and any breastfeeding in the first 6 months of age, as recommended by the WHO and the American Academy of Pediatrics.[50]

## CONGENITAL MALFORMATIONS IN THE OFFSPRING OF DIABETIC MOTHER

Maternal hyperglycemia as the major cause mediating teratogenicity, regardless of its cause, is responsible for increased rate of birth defects in the offspring. The rate of birth defects increases linearly with the degree of maternal hyperglycemia. Prenatal glycemic control is effective mean to reduce birth defects in offspring from diabetic pregnancies, but cannot reduce the incidence of birth defects to the rate that is seen in the nondiabetic population.[4] Studies in animal models have revealed that diabetes in pregnancy induces oxidative stress, which activates cellular stress signaling leading to dysregulation of gene expression and excess apoptosis in the target organs, including the neural tube and embryonic heart.[4] Activation of the apoptosis signal-regulating kinase 1 (ASK1)–forkhead transcription factor 3a (FOXO3a)–caspase 8 pathway causes apoptosis in the developing neural tube leading to neural tube defects (NTDs). *ASK1* activates the c-Jun-N-Terminal kinase 1/2 (JNK1/2), which leads to activation of the unfolded protein response and endoplasmic reticulum (ER) stress. Deletion of the *ASK1* gene, the *JNK1* gene, or the *JNK2* gene, or inhibition of ER stress by 4-Phenylbutyric acid nullifies diabetes-induced apoptosis and reduces the formation of NTDs.[4] Antioxidants, such as thioredoxin, which inhibits the ASK1-FOXO3a-caspase 8 pathway or ER stress inhibitors, may prevent pregestational diabetes-induced birth defects.[4]

Not many studies (only 17 studies out of 3,488 abstracts) were found to be investigating the risk of congenital malformations in pregnancies with gestational diabetes.[51] A higher risk of major congenital malformations was observed in offspring of women with gestational diabetes with the following RR/odds ratios (ORs) and 95% CI: RR 1.16 (1.07–1.25) in cohort studies and OR 1.4 (1.22–1.62) in case–control studies. The risk of major congenital malformations was much higher in offspring of women with pregestational diabetes mellitus (PGDM) than in those of the reference group: RR 2.66 (2.04–3.47) in cohort studies and OR 4.7 (3.01–6.95) in the single case–control study.[51] Pregestational diabetes mellitus is associated with a wide range of anomalies in almost any fetal organ. According to some published data, women with PGDM have two- to ninefold higher risk of having babies with birth defects, with a prevalence of birth defects of 2.7–18.6%, compared with the healthy population, having a prevalence of birth defects of 2–3%.[4] Although any birth defect can be associated with PGDM, more anomalies are seen in the cardiovascular, central nervous, and skeletal systems. Caudal regression syndrome with femoral shortening and sacral agenesis is rare congenital malformation almost exclusively associated with PGDM.[52]

Congenital anomalies of the kidney and urinary tract (CAKUT) are among the major reasons in young adults needing renal replacement therapy, but there is a little extensive assessment of their incidence and risk factors. Of 1,603,794 newborns registered between 2004 and 2014 in Taiwan, 668 infants were reported to have CAKUT.[53] The incidence of CAKUT was approximately 4.2 per 10,000 births. The adjusted OR for CAKUT in newborns associated with maternal gestational diabetes was OR, 2.22, 95% CI, 1.06–4.67.[53] Infants of a mother with gestational diabetes were more likely to have congenital anomalies, small gestational age (<37 weeks) and low-birth weight.[53] In another study, 945 case-patients with CAKUT and 4,725 controls (matched for gestational age, sex, and birth year) were identified.[54] Maternal PGDM occurred in 39 (4.1%) of the CAKUT group and 111 (2.3%) controls (P = 0.002), whereas GDM occurred in 40 (4.2%) of the CAKUT group and 157 (3.3%) controls (P = 0.2)—not statistically significant.[54] A multivariate logistic regression model revealed that PGDM was associated with CAKUT (OR, 1.67; 95% CI, 1.14–2.46), whereas GDM was not (OR, 1.29; 95% CI, 0.90–1.85).[54] The association between CAKUT and LGA suggests that poor glycemic control before and in pregnancy increases risk of CAKUT.[54]

Prepregnancy care for women with pregestational type 1 or type 2 diabetes mellitus is effective in decreasing the rates of congenital malformations, perinatal mortality, and in reducing maternal HbA1c in the first trimester of pregnancy.[55]

Treatment of pregestational diabetes with metformin, which crosses the placenta is increasing the risk of its possible adverse fetal effects.[56,57] The available data suggest that metformin exposure during the first trimester is not associated with increased prevalence of major congenital malformations; that metformin reduces the risk of early pregnancy loss, preeclampsia, preterm delivery, and GDM in women with polycystic ovarian disease.[56] Metformin treatment is associated with at least comparable benefits relative to insulin treatment in women with mild GDM, and that child neurodevelopmental outcomes at the age of 1.5–2.5 years are comparable after gestational exposure to metformin and insulin.[56,57] In another paper investigating use of metformin in obese and women with polycystic ovary syndrome, they revealed that the use of metformin throughout pregnancy reduces the rates of early pregnancy loss and preterm labor and protects against fetal growth restriction, while there have been no demonstrable teratogenic effects, intrauterine deaths or developmental delays with the use of metformin.[58]

# NEURODEVELOPMENTAL AND PSYCHIATRIC OUTCOME OF THE NEWBORNS FROM DIABETIC PREGNANCIES

Besides hyperglycemia, which is a potential major teratogenic factor in the offspring from diabetic pregnancies, hypoglycemia is another threat sporadically connected with impaired child neurodevelopment.[59] According to some authors risk factors for neonatal hypoglycemic brain injury could be—gestational age less than or equal to 36 weeks; birth weight less than small for gestational age (especially infants below the third percentile); infants born to diabetic mothers and infants with Beckwith-Wiedemann syndrome or Rh hemolytic disease; islet cell dysregulation syndrome, insulinoma; perinatal asphyxia; impact of mothers' drugs, such as beta-blockers; neonatal septicemia; and congenital metabolic disorders like deficiency of enzymes for glycogenolysis, gluconeogenesis, or beta-oxidation of fatty acids.[59]

Criteria for neonatal hypoglycemic brain injury are not explicitly determined and vary from author to author. In one study, the following diagnostic criteria for neonatal hypoglycemic brain injury have been proposed—whole blood glucose less than or equal to 2.0 mmol/L; history of severe hypoglycemia (0–1.7 mmol/L) or obvious hypoglycemia-related clinical manifestations at admission; symptoms of central nervous system disorder like neonatal convulsions in course of severe hypoglycemia, which has been corrected by intravenous glucose application; neuroimaging (mostly magnetic resonance imaging) changes in the brain caused by hypoglycemia, once other conditions causing brain injury like intracranial bleeding, congenital malformations of the brain, intracranial infections, and congenital metabolic disorders have been excluded.[60,61] Besides normoglycemia, it has been speculated that diet enriched with docosahexaenoic acid (DHA) in pregnancy may be linked with undisturbed infant neurodevelopment.[62] DHA (omega-3 fatty acid) is a structural component of neural tissue playing an important role in brain development.[62] Besides already mentioned decreased transplacental maternofetal iron transfer in women with diabetes, DHA transfer is reduced as well, although evidence of mechanisms explaining altered maternofetal DHA transfer is limited.[62] Further research is necessary to evaluate the role of peroxisome proliferator-activated receptors in modulating placental fatty acid binding and maternofetal DHA transfer.[62] It is of some importance for everyday clinical practice to supplement DHA in the diet of obstetric diabetic patients.[62]

Potential brain injury with short- and long-term neurodevelopmental consequences is the major reason to manage low-blood glucose concentrations in the patients most at risk for asymptomatic hypoglycemia like those born late-preterm, LGA, small for gestational age, or growth restricted, and those born following a pregnancy complicated by diabetes mellitus.[63] It is estimated that 15% of low-risk newborn babies and 50% of high-risk neonates are affected by neonatal hypoglycemia.[64] The first step in the treatment of neonatal hypoglycemia usually involves additional feeding (breastfeeding first, and then if the breast milk is unavailable infant formula), and frequent admission to NICU for intravenous dextrose, which may be costly and inhibiting the establishment of breastfeeding. Prevention of neonatal hypoglycemia would be desirable, but there are currently no strategies, beyond early feeding, for prevention of neonatal hypoglycemia. Application of 40% dextrose buccal gel (200 mg/kg) in the dose of 0.5 mL/kg is safe and effective in the treatment of neonatal hypoglycemia, decreasing the admission rate to the NICU due to neonatal hypoglycemia from 10–6% and rise in blood glucose concentration following dextrose gel by 0.4 mmol/L.[64,65]

There were no significant differences between children with neonatal normoglycemia and hypoglycemia (plasma glucose <2.2 mmol/L 1 hour after birth or <2.5 mmol/L, subsequently) in Denver developmental scale scores and child behavior checklist scores, and total intelligence quotient (IQ) did not differ between hypoglycemic and normoglycemic children.[66] There were no differences in any of the test scores between hypoglycemic children who had and who had not been treated with intravenous glucose.[66] Authors concluded that transient mild hypoglycemia in healthy, term LGA newborns does not appear to be harmful to psychomotor development at the age of 4 years.[66]

It seems that the situation with the children born from diabetic pregnancies is quite different due to maternal and fetal metabolic dysfunction leading to diminished iron stores, a metabolism-placental perfusion mismatch, increased free fatty acid (FFA), increased lactic acidosis, and potential hypoxia, leading to the suggestion from empirical research that such hostile environment can adversely affect neurodevelopment of the offspring leading to lower general intelligence, language impairments, attention weaknesses, impulsivity, and behavioral problems.[67,68] Therefore, appropriate glucose control during pregnancy, which may help to reduce the neurodevelopmental effects of gestational diabetes, is important and should be looking for by clinicians evaluating children with developmental learning or cognitive dysfunction.[67]

Besides GDM, maternal socioeconomic status is importantly associated with the risk for attention-deficit hyperactivity disorder (ADHD) in children. Nomura and ass. found that there was an association between higher prevalence rate of GDM with lower socioeconomic status.[69] In the same study, both maternal GDM and low-socioeconomic status were associated with an approximately two fold increased risk for ADHD at the age 6 years.[69] The risk for ADHD increased over 14-fold when children were exposed to both GDM and low-socioeconomic status. Besides that, children exposed to both GDM and low-socioeconomic status demonstrated impaired neurobehavioral functioning, including lower IQ, poorer language, behavioral and emotional functioning.[69]

In the recently published meta-analysis of 7,698 references reviewed, 12 studies involving 6,140 infants met inclusion criteria and contributed to meta-analysis of children (1–2 years) of diabetic mothers who had significantly lower scores of mental and psychomotor development compared to control infants.[68] Diabetes during pregnancy could be associated with decreased IQ scores in school-age children, although studies showed significant heterogeneity.[68] The association between maternal diabetes and deleterious effects on mental/psychomotor development and overall intellectual function in the offspring must be taken with caution because the results are based on observational cohorts and a direct causal influence of intrauterine hyperglycemia remains uncertain.[68]

Interestingly, in the recently published population-based cohort study from Israel, the association between in utero exposure to GDM and neuropsychiatric disorders and possible association with autistic spectrum disorder has been found.[70] During the study period 231,271 deliveries met the inclusion criteria; 5.4% of the births were to mothers diagnosed with GDM (n = 12,642), of these 4.3% had gestational diabetes type A1 (n = 10,076) and 1.1% had gestational diabetes type A2 (n = 2,566).[70] During the follow-up period, a significant linear association was noted between the severity of gestational diabetes (no gestational diabetes, GDM A1, GDM A2) and neuropsychiatric disease of the offspring (1.02% vs. 1.36% vs. 1.68%, respectively, P <0.001).[70] Maternal GDM was found to be an independent risk factor for long-term neuropsychiatric disease of the offspring [GDM A1 (adjusted OR, 1.83; 95% CI, 1.53–2.19) and GDM A2 (adjusted OR, 1.64; 95% CI, 1.18–2.27)].[70] Their findings also point to a possible association between in utero exposure to GDM and autistic spectrum disorder of the offspring (adjusted OR, 4.44; 95% CI, 1.55–12.69).[70]

## CONCLUSION

In the last years due to quick environmental and dietary changes, social and economic development, and many other known and unknown reasons, the mankind is faced with the changing pathology during pregnancy.[71] Currently, 60 million women of reproductive age worldwide have diabetes mellitus, and it has been estimated that this number will double by 2030.[4] Many potentially deleterious effects of diabetes mellitus in pregnancy like hyperglycemia, hypoglycemia, hyperinsulinism, diminished iron stores, a metabolism-placental perfusion mismatch, decreased DHA, increased FFA, increased lactic acidosis, and potential hypoxia can affect the mother and her offspring. Healthcare systems should be prepared to react properly in order to prevent consequences for the mother and her offspring.

## REFERENCES

1. Ferrara A. Increasing prevalence of gestational diabetes mellitus. Diabetes Care. 2007;30:S141-6.
2. Hashimoto K, Koga M. Indicators of glycemic control in patients with gestational diabetes mellitus and pregnant women with diabetes mellitus. World J Diabetes. 2015;6:1045-56.
3. Macaulay S, Dunger DB, Norris SA. Gestational diabetes mellitus in Africa: a systematic review. PLoS ONE. 2014;9:e97871.
4. Gabbay-Benziv R, Reece EA, Wang F, et al. Birth defects in pregestational diabetes: defect range, glycemic threshold and pathogenesis. World J Diabetes. 2015;6:481-8.
5. Catalano PM, Hauguel-De Mouzon S. Is it time to revisit the Pedersen hypothesis in the face of the obesity epidemic? Am J Obstet Gynecol. 2011;204:479-87.
6. Pedersen J. Diabetes and pregnancy; blood sugar of newborn infants during fasting and glucose administration. Ugeskr Laeger. 1952;114:685.
7. The HAPO Study Cooperative Research Group. Hyperglycemia and Adverse Pregnancy Outcome (HAPO) Study. Associations with neonatal anthropometrics. Diabetes. 2009;58:453-9.
8. Ashwal E, Hod M. Gestational diabetes mellitus: Where are we now? Clin Chim Acta. 2015;451: 14-20.
9. Barker DJ. The origins of the developmental origins theory. J Intern Med. 2007;261:412-7.
10. Gillman MW, Barker D, Bier D, et al. Meeting report on the 3rd International Congress on Developmental Origins of Health and Disease (DOHaD). Pediatr Res. 2007;61:625-9.
11. Mitanchez D, Yzydorczyk C, Siddeek B, et al. The offspring of the diabetic mother—short- and long-term implications. Best Pract Res Clin Obstet Gynaecol. 2015;29:256-69.
12. Yessoufou A, Moutairou K. Maternal diabetes in pregnancy: early and long-term outcomes on the offspring and the concept of "metabolic memory". Exp Diabetes Res. 2011;2011:218598.
13. Wadhwa PD, Buss C, Entringer S, et al. Developmental origins of health and disease: brief history of the approach and current focus on epigenetic mechanisms. Semin Reprod Med. 2009;27:358-68.
14. Kitzmiller JL. Sweet success with diabetes. The development of insulin therapy and glycemic control for pregnancy. Diabetes Care. 1993;16:107-21.
15. Cordero L, Treuer SH, Landon MB, et al. Management of infants of diabetic mothers. Arch Pediatr Adolesc Med. 1998;152:249-54.
16. Lloreda-García JM, Sevilla-Denia S, Rodríguez-Sánchez A, et al. Perinatal outcome of macrosomic infants born to diabetic versus non-diabetic mothers. Endocrinol Nutr. 2016;63:409-13.
17. Sugawara D, Maruyama A, Imanishi T, et al. Complications in infants of diabetic mothers related to glycated albumin and hemoglobin levels during pregnancy. Pediatr Neonatol. 2016;57:496-500.
18. Meek CL, Lewis HB, Patient C, et al. Diagnosis of gestational diabetes mellitus: falling through the net. Diabetologia. 2015;58:2003-12.
19. Boghossian NS, Hansen NI, Bell EF, et al. Outcomes of extremely preterm infants born to insulin-dependent diabetic mothers. Pediatrics. 2016;137:pii: e20153424.
20. Tunay ZÖ, Özdemir Ö, Acar DE, et al. Maternal diabetes as an independent risk factor for retinopathy of prematurity in infants with birth weight of 1500 g or more. Am J Ophthalmol. 2016;168: 201-6.
21. Lasheen AE, Abdelbasit OB, Seidahmed MZ, et al. Infants of diabetic mothers. A cohort study. Saudi Med J. 2014;35:572-7.

22. Gauster M, Desoye G, Tötsch M, et al. The placenta and gestational diabetes mellitus. Curr Diab Rep. 2012;12:16-23.
23. Li HP, Chen X, Li MQ. Gestational diabetes induces chronic hypoxia stress and excessive inflammatory response in murine placenta. Int J Clin Exp Pathol. 2013;6:650-9.
24. Viteri OA, Dinis J, Roman T, et al. Timing of medically indicated delivery in diabetic pregnancies: a perspective on current evidence-based recommendations. Am J Perinatol. 2016;33:821-5.
25. Taricco E, Radaelli T, Rossi G, et al. Effects of gestational diabetes on fetal oxygen and glucose levels in vivo. BJOG. 2009;116:1729-35.
26. Treviño-Alanís M, Ventura-Juárez J, Hernández-Piñero J, et al. Delayed lung maturation of foetus of diabetic mother rats develop with a diminish, but without changes in the proportion of type I and II pneumocytes, and decreased expression of protein D-associated surfactant factor. Anat Histol Embryol. 2009;38:169-76.
27. Hrabovski I, Milašinović L, Bogavac M, et al. Cardiorespiratory disorders of infants of diabetic mothers. Srp Arh Celok Lek. 2015;143:567-72.
28. Persson M, Fadl H. Perinatal outcome in relation to fetal sex in offspring to mothers with pregestational and gestational diabetes—a population-based study. Diabet Med. 2014;31:1047-54.
29. Joutsi-Korhonen L, Aitokallio-Tallberg A, Halmesmäki E, et al. Amniotic lamellar body counts determined with the Sysmex XE-2100 analyzer to predict fetal lung maturity during diabetic and other complicated pregnancies. Scand J Clin Lab Invest. 2010;70:358-63.
30. Stanley CA. Perspective on the genetics and diagnosis of congenital hyperinsulinism disorders. J Clin Endocrinol Metab. 2016;101:815-26.
31. Huang T, Kelly A, Becker SA, et al. Hypertrophic cardiomyopathy in neonates with congenital hyperinsulinism. Arch Dis Child Fetal Neonatal Ed. 2013;98:F351-4.
32. Abu-Sulaiman RM, Subaih B. Congenital heart disease in infants of diabetic mothers: echocardiographic study. Pediatr Cardiol. 2004;25:137-40.
33. Hăşmăşanu MG, Bolboacă SD, Matyas M, et al. Clinical and echocardiographic findings in newborns of diabetic mothers. Acta Clin Croat. 2015;54:458-66.
34. Al-Biltagi M, Tolba OA, Rowisha MA, et al. Speckle tracking and myocardial tissue imaging in infant of diabetic mother with gestational and pregestational diabetes. Pediatr Cardiol. 2015;36:445-53.
35. Welters A, Lerch C, Kummer S, et al. Long-term medical treatment in congenital hyperinsulinism: a descriptive analysis in a large cohort of patients from different clinical centers. Orphanet J Rare Dis. 2015;10:150.
36. Mongiovì M, Fesslova V, Fazio G, et al. Diagnosis and prognosis of fetal cardiomyopathies: a review. Curr Pharm Des. 2010;16:2929-34.
37. Logan KM, Gale C, Hyde MJ, et al. Diabetes in pregnancy and infant adiposity: systematic review and meta-analysis. Arch Dis Child Fetal Neonatal Ed. 2017;102:F65-F72.
38. Starling AP, Brinton JT, Glueck DH, et al. Associations of maternal BMI and gestational weight gain with neonatal adiposity in the Healthy Start study. Am J Clin Nutr. 2015;101:302-9.
39. Malinowska-Polubiec A, Romejko-Wolniewicz E, Szostak O, et al. Shoulder dystocia in diabetic and non-diabetic pregnancies. Neuro Endocrinol Lett. 2014;35:733-40.
40. Gunderson EP, Hurston SR, Dewey KG, et al. The study of women, infant feeding and type 2 diabetes after GDM pregnancy and growth of their offspring (SWIFT Offspring study): prospective design, methodology and baseline characteristics. BMC Pregnancy Childbirth. 2015;15:150.
41. Linder N, Lahat Y, Kogan A, et al. Macrosomic newborns of non-diabetic mothers: anthropometric measurements and neonatal complications. Arch Dis Child Fetal Neonatal Ed. 2014;99:F353-8.
42. de Onis M, Garza C, Onyango AW, et al. WHO Child Growth Standards. Acta Paediatr. 2006;95:1-104. [online] Available from: http://www.who.int/childgrowth/standards/Acta_95_S450.pdf?ua=1. [Accessed August, 2017].
43. Dewey KG, Heinig MJ, Nommsen LA, et al. Breast-fed infants are leaner than formula-fed infants at 1 y of age: the DARLING study. Am J Clin Nutr. 1993;57:140-5.

44. Dewey KG, Peerson JM, Brown KH, et al. Growth of breast-fed infants deviates from current reference data: a pooled analysis of US, Canadian, and European data sets. World Health Organization Working Group on Infant Growth. Pediatrics. 1995;96:495-503.

45. Grunewald M, Hellmuth C, Demmelmair H, et al. Excessive weight gain during full breast-feeding. Ann Nutr Metab. 2014;64:271-5.

46. Whitaker RC, Dietz WH. Role of the prenatal environment in the development of obesity. J Pediatr. 1998;132:768-76.

47. Touger L, Looker HC, Krakoff J, et al. Early growth in offspring of diabetic mothers. Diabetes Care. 2005;28:585-9.

48. Vohr BR, McGarvey ST. Growth patterns of large-for-gestational-age and appropriate-for-gestational-age infants of gestational diabetic mothers and control mothers at age 1 year. Diabetes Care. 1997;20:1066-72.

49. Schaefer-Graf UM, Pawliczak J, Passow D, et al. Birth weight and parental BMI predict overweight in children from mothers with gestational diabetes. Diabetes Care. 2005;28:1745-50.

50. Trout KK, Averbuch T, Barowski M. Promoting breastfeeding among obese women and women with gestational diabetes mellitus. Curr Diab Rep. 2011;11:7-12.

51. Balsells M, García-Patterson A, Gich I, et al. Major congenital malformations in women with gestational diabetes mellitus: a systematic review and meta-analysis. Diabetes Metab Res Rev. 2012;28:252-7.

52. Hay WW Jr. Care of the infant of the diabetic mother. Curr Diab Rep. 2012;12:4-15.

53. Tain YL, Luh H, Lin CY, et al. Incidence and risks of congenital anomalies of kidney and urinary tract in newborns: a population-based case-control study in Taiwan. Medicine (Baltimore). 2016;95:e2659.

54. Dart AB, Ruth CA, Sellers EA, et al. Maternal diabetes mellitus and congenital anomalies of the kidney and urinary tract (CAKUT) in the child. Am J Kidney Dis. 2015;65:684-91.

55. Wahabi HA, Alzeidan RA, Esmaeil SA. Pre-pregnancy care for women with pre-gestational diabetes mellitus: a systematic review and meta-analysis. BMC Public Health. 2012;12:792.

56. Andrade C. Major malformation risk, pregnancy outcomes, and neurodevelopmental outcomes associated with metformin use during pregnancy. J Clin Psychiatry. 2016;77:e411-4.

57. Singh AK, Singh R. Metformin in gestational diabetes: an emerging contender. Indian J Endocrinol Metab. 2015;19:236-44.

58. Lautatzis ME, Goulis DG, Vrontakis M. Efficacy and safety of metformin during pregnancy in women with gestational diabetes mellitus or polycystic ovary syndrome: a systematic review. Metabolism. 2013;62:1522-34.

59. Straussman S, Levitsky LL. Neonatal hypoglycemia. Curr Opin Endocrinol Diabetes Obes. 2010;17:20-4.

60. Mao J, Chen LY, Fu JH, et al. Clinical evaluation of neonatal hypoglycemic brain injury demonstrated by serial MRIs. Zhongguo Dang Dai Er Ke Za Zhi. 2008;10:115-20.

61. Su J, Wang L. Research advances in neonatal hypoglycemic brain injury. Transl Pediatr. 2012;1:108-15.

62. Judge MP, Casavant SG, Dias JA, et al. Reduced DHA transfer in diabetic pregnancies: mechanistic basis and long-term neurodevelopmental implications. Nutr Rev. 2016;74:411-20.

63. Rozance PJ, Hay WW Jr. New approaches to management of neonatal hypoglycemia. Matern Health Neonatol Perinatol. 2016;2:3.

64. Harding JE, Hegarty JE, Crowther CA, et al. Randomised trial of neonatal hypoglycaemia prevention with oral dextrose gel (hPOD): study protocol. BMC Pediatr. 2015;15:120.

65. Weston PJ, Harris DL, Battin M, et al. Oral dextrose gel for the treatment of hypoglycaemia in newborn infants. Cochrane Database Syst Rev. 2016;5:CD011027.

66. Brand PL, Molenaar NL, Kaaijk C, et al. Neurodevelopmental outcome of hypoglycaemia in healthy, large for gestational age, term newborns. Arch Dis Child. 2005;90:78-81.

67. Perna R, Loughan AR, Le J, et al. Gestational diabetes: long-term central nervous system developmental and cognitive sequelae. Appl Neuropsychol Child. 2015;4:217-20.
68. Camprubi Robles M, Campoy C, Garcia Fernandez L, et al. Maternal diabetes and cognitive performance in the offspring: a systematic review and meta-analysis. PLoS One. 2015;10:e0142583.
69. Nomura Y, Marks DJ, Grossman B, et al. Exposure to gestational diabetes mellitus and low socioeconomic status: effects on neurocognitive development and risk of attention-deficit/hyperactivity disorder in offspring. Arch Pediatr Adolesc Med. 2012;166:337-43.
70. Nahum Sacks K, Friger M, Shoham-Vardi I, et al. Prenatal exposure to gestational diabetes mellitus as an independent risk factor for long-term neuropsychiatric morbidity of the offspring. Am J Obstet Gynecol. 2016;215:380.e1-7.
71. Kurjak A. First 10 years of the International Academy of Perinatal Medicine—which lessons we have learned and what are future challenges. J Perinat Med. 2016;44:733-5.

# Chapter 8

# Artificial Maturation of Fetus in all Kinds of Diabetes

*Miroslava Gojnic, Milan Perovic, Igor V Pantic, Badreldeen Ahmed*

## INTRODUCTION

Birth, the emergence and separation of offspring from the body of the mother, is the event that divides our intrauterine from our postnatal life and brings dramatic changes in our body. Separation from placenta deprives the offspring from the former gas exchange, nutrient uptake, waste elimination, thermoregulation, protection against infection and hormone supply.[1] Therefore, in order to meet these future needs, fetal organs and tissues go through maturational changes in late pregnancy.[1] The lungs mature structurally and functionally, becoming distensible and capable of coping with high surface tension when air comes into the alveoli with the first breath. In the liver, glycogen stores and gluconeogenesis is commenced to meet the demands for glucose until feeding begins. There is an increase in the production of thyroid hormone, vital for the body's metabolism, function of heart and digestive system, control of the muscles, brain development and the maintenance of bones. Furthermore, the intensification in the synthesis of catecholamines has the role in preparation for the sharp increase in metabolic rate and thermogenesis associated with breathing and the cold environment.

Preterm delivery is the most important issue in perinatology due to several facts. The most important one refers to prematurity as the leading cause of death in children under the age of five. Furthermore, the prevalence of preterm birth is high, with more than 1 in 10 babies born premature.[2] Therefore, this chapter is dedicated to artificial acceleration of fetal lungs in imminent or initiated preterm delivery, with emphasis on modality treatments of those pregnancies complicated with different types of diabetes.

## PHYSIOLOGY PROCESSES IN FETAL LUNG MATURATION

Maturational events in fetus during late gestation are essential for neonatal survival and health. These events are regulated by endogenous glucocorticosteroids, primarily by cortisol, but also by corticosterone. They induce synthesis of a number of enzymes that are without or with a little function during intrauterine life, but that are nevertheless crucial for life after birth.[1] Glucocorticoids achieve their roles in fetal maturation by bonding to glucocorticoid receptors (GRs, or the type 2 receptors), located in cells of various target organs and tissues. They are playing important role in functional maturing of those organs that are essential for survival of newborn, such as liver, heart, kidney, lung, skin and gut. Physiological production of glucocorticoids in fetus is firmly controlled, it starts at 28th week of gestation and increases significantly shortly before birth. Markedly increased levels of fetal glucocorticoids in late gestation act through GRs in order to elicit the essential maturation of fetal organs. Glucocorticoids modify gene expressions responsible for different important processes. While glucocorticoids are accountable for processes of proteolysis and lipolysis in some organs and some periods of life,[3] they are also responsible for opposite processes in different targets and periods of time, such as biosynthesis of proteins and phospholipids and the appearance of surfactant production in the fetal lung.[4] In that respect, glucocorticoid activity has the most important role in adjusting fetal and postnatal lung development.[5]

There are several mechanisms of glucocorticoid action in the acceleration of fetal pulmonary maturation, such as improving pulmonary compliance, increasing alveolar surfactant and expanding maximal lung volume.[4] One mechanism is taking the action through the improvement in fetal lung mechanics. Experiment conducted on fetal sheep revealed that treatment with betamethasone instigated improved dynamic thoracic compliance and ventilatory efficiency index and doubled up lung gas volume when compared to control group.[6] Other mechanism refers to upsurge in surfactant proteins and lipids. Gene transcription-mediated action of prenatal glucocorticoid stimulation of surfactant proteins B and C is acknowledged in human fetuses.[7] All these dramatic maturational events are regulated by cortisol as there are numerous others in most organ systems that contribute to neonatal health but on which survival is less dependent. This knowledge is used in pharmacological manipulation of these systems before birth and has made a substantial contribution in decreasing consequences of preterm birth and in improving neonatal and general postnatal health. While the major form of active glucocorticoid in human beings is cortisol, in clinical practice, betamethasone and dexamethasone are main glucocorticoids used for acceleration of fetal lung maturation.[8]

Furthermore, labor has the significant role in fetal lung maturation. Vaginal squeeze of fetus during labor causes physiological catecholamine surge[9,10] and facilitates alveolar fluid drainage.[11,12] This knowledge is of great importance for those women who are delivered by planned elective cesarean section. Therefore, those women are at higher risk for respiratory distress syndrome (RDS) even if delivered at term. Glucocorticoids seem to increase the number and function of sodium channels as well as the sensitivity to catecholamine and thyroid hormones, providing a justification for their exogenous use in planned cesarean deliveries.[9-12] Having in mind that the women with pregnancies complicated with diabetes are at risk for cesarean section for several reasons (macrosomic baby, polyhydramnios, increased risk for fetal hypoxia during pregnancy and labor), all of this physiological processes and issues have to be taken into account during the management of these high risk pregnancies.

## PATHOPHYSIOLOGICAL PROCESSES THAT INFLUENCE FETAL LUNG MATURATION IN PREGNANCIES COMPLICATED BY DIABETES

Fetal pulmonary maturation is delayed in pregnancies complicated by diabetes. This observation stemmed from the results of numerous studies that evaluated maturation of fetal lung by measurements of biochemical indicators of pulmonary maturity, such as lecithin to sphingomyelin ratio, phosphatidylglycerol (PG) and by the occurrence of hyaline membrane disease even in term gestations.

A case–control study performed with 295 pregnant women with diabetes and 590 control subjects was performed to conclude whether there are differences in the timing of the appearance of various amniotic fluid fetal pulmonary phospholipids in normal and diabetic pregnancy.[13] Gestational age-matched amniocentesis specimens were evaluated for lecithin/sphingomyelin (L/S) ratio, phosphatidylinositol (PI), and PG composition. Stratification of pregnant women with diabetes was done according to type of diabetes, degree of blood glucose control, and birth percentile of the neonate. The beginning of production of PG was delayed from 35.9 +/– 1.1 weeks (controls) to 38.7 +/– 0.9 weeks (overt diabetics) and 37.3 +/– 1.0 weeks for gestational diabetes mellitus (P <0.001). While the authors did not find the delay in PG synthesis associated to level of maternal glucose control,[13] the outcomes of a different study indicate that poorly controlled maternal glucose levels are associated with delayed appearance of PG in diabetic pregnancies.[14] In the study performed on 261 diabetic pregnancies with good glycemic control and 360 diabetic pregnancies with poor glycemic control, the amniotic fluid was inspected for PG whose presence is considered as indicator of lung maturity. The study results demonstrated that poorly controlled maternal glucose levels are associated with delayed appearance of amniotic fluid PG in diabetic pregnancies.[14] Furthermore, when stratified by gestational age, the risk of absence of PG was significantly higher in the poor glycemic control group (odds ratio 1.83, confidence interval 1.19-2.84), therefore concluding that poorly controlled maternal glucose levels are associated with delayed appearance of PG in pregnancies complicated by diabetes.[14]

All these findings were also confirmed by experimental studies performed on diabetes-induced animals. One experimental study performed on rats has demonstrated a delay in alveolarization of the offspring of the diabetic group compared to control groups.[15] This was confirmed by transmission electron microscopy of lung biopsy specimens. Furthermore, fetuses of the diabetic group revealed a postponement in lung histogenesis and in differentiation of the type 2 pneumocyte cells. Moreover, less quantity of protein D associated to surfactant in streptozotocin-induced pregnant diabetic rats was found.[15]

## SYNTHETIC CORTICOSTEROIDS FOR ANTENATAL THERAPY AND PROPHYLAXIS

In general, there are two major groups of indication for the use of synthetic corticosteroids during pregnancy. The first encompasses all maternal diseases or other pregnancy related problems, such as rheumatological problems, systemic lupus erythematosus, inflammatory bowel disease, Addison's disease and idiopathic thrombocytopenic purpura. For these reasons, those corticosteroids that are crossing placenta in small amounts should be used. In contrast, in the second group where the target of antenatal corticosteroids (ACS) is the fetus (either for treatment of fetal congenital adrenal hyperplasia or for acceleration of fetal lung maturation), those corticosteroids that are crossing the placenta freely (betamethasone and dexamethasone) should be used.[16]

Glucocorticoids are crucial for the shift from fetal to neonatal life. In cases of premature birth, antenatally given artificial corticoids should replace physiological increase of endogenous glucocorticoids (example cortisol) which would not take place due premature termination of pregnancy.[17,18] Pioneers of ACS treatment for women at risk of preterm birth, Liggins and Howie, performed studies firstly on experimental animals[17] but very soon these studies were followed by clinical trials and both types of studies were united in the conclusion.[18] Application of ACS is effective treatment in preventing neonatal consequences of premature birth, such as RDS, neonatal death and intraventricular hemorrhage.[19] The first official endorsement for ACS use by some renowned institution or professional society was from the National Institutes of Health. In the Consensus Development Conference Statement in 1995 brought by the National Institutes of Health says that use of betamethasone or dexamethasone in women at high risk for preterm delivery prevents RDS in neonates.[20] The decision regarding the choice of synthetic corticosteroids for accelerated fetal maturation was done after meta-analysis of randomized clinical trials that establish betamethasone and dexamethasone to be similarly effective in preventing RDS.[21] However, level III evidence derived from a large observational study suggested that antenatal use of betamethasone is related with a reduced possibility of cystic periventricular leukomalacia among premature newborns born at 24–31 gestational week.[22] Conversely, this finding was not found with dexamethasone treatment.[22] Therefore, the Scientific Advisory Committee of Royal College of Obstetricians and Gynaecologists endorses betamethasone as the steroid of choice to enhance fetal lung maturation.[4]

It has been known for many decades that pregnancy complicated with diabetes is independently related with higher risk of neonatal RDS.[23] Newborns of mothers with pregestational or gestational diabetes mellitus who are born premature may be predisposed to pulmonary immaturity at more advanced periods of gestation than newborns of nondiabetic mothers. Therefore, the requisite for ACS therapy is expected to be greater in the presence of pregnancy-accompanied diabetes.

## Indications for Antenatal Prophylactic Administration of Synthetic Corticosteroids

The purpose of antenatal prophylactic administration of corticosteroids is to reduce the incidence of RDS by speeding up fetal lung maturation. This treatment before 35 weeks of gestation is intended for preterm premature rupture of membranes, threatened preterm labor and antepartum hemorrhage.[24,25] Although the use of ACS after 34 weeks is controversial, recent position statements of renowned professional and scientific associations and recent meta-analysis of randomized controlled trials recommend ACS for women at risk of late premature delivery,[26] and for all women with a planned elective cesarean section prior to 38 weeks of gestation.[24,27]

## IMPLICATIONS OF ANTENATAL CORTICOSTEROIDS FOR FETAL LUNG MATURATION IN WOMEN WITH DIABETES

Pregnancies complicated by diabetes are at higher risk for spontaneous and elective preterm deliveries (either by cesarean section or per vias naturalis) compared to the pregnancies in general population of women,[28] and therefore are at higher need for ACS treatment for accelerating fetal maturation. Despite some concerns regarding ACS usage in diabetic patients, the indications for ACS are determined by perinatal and obstetric aspects rather than medical issues, and recommendations for this treatment stay the same regardless of glycemic status. However, this part of the chapter will discuss special considerations and patient monitoring that have to be taken in pregnant women who are treated with ACS.

The use of ACS has several adverse maternal effects and the most significant are altered glucose tolerance and adrenal suppression. Fetal lung maturation with ACS affects maternal glucose metabolism and the extent of that influence is dependent of basic maternal metabolic condition and with the number of fetuses in womb. While ACS in healthy women with singleton pregnancies carries insignificant degree of alteration of maternal fasting plasma glucose levels that are remaining within a normal range, ACS in healthy women with multiple pregnancies or in women with impaired glucose metabolism brings the elevation of glycemic levels above normal ranges.[29] The best illustration of these facts are the findings of Refuerzo et al. who found that after ACS administration, increase of glucose levels in women with gestational diabetes was up to 3 times higher compared to healthy women.[30] Therefore, glucose intolerance and diabetes are conditions where the use of ACS for fetal lung maturation should be done with special considerations, since the medical treatment with ACS caries the risk of maternal hyperglycemia.[30-32]

In order to evaluate the timing and the extent of increase of blood glucose values after administration of ACS, several studies have been performed.[30-32] All studies demonstrated the increase of these levels, but they have conflicting results regarding the timing of the highest increase of glycemic levels. In the study of Itoh et al., women with gestational diabetes who have received betamethasone intramuscularly have been monitored and evaluation of maternal glycemia and insulin dosage needed shown that the insulin dosage needed for glycemic control gradually increased, reaching a maximum at 10 hours after the betamethasone application and decreasing at the pretreatment level 24 hours after the application of ACS.[31] Jolley et al. compared blood glucose levels after the treatment with ACS in women with and without diabetes. Their findings demonstrated earlier attainment of the highest increase of blood glucose values in women with diabetes compared to healthy women. The highest mean blood glucose level occurred at 6 hours after ACS application in women with diabetes and at 30 hours in women without diabetes.[32] The results of study of Refuerzo et al. are to a certain extent different. They confirmed that the return to the pretreatment level of glycemia happens 24 hours after the treatment, but the highest blood glucose levels occur at 20 hours after ACS application.[30]

Bearing in mind that the use of medications for delaying premature birth are given in order to allow enough time for ACS to take action, we need to address the issue of the tocolytic medicine selection as regards their effect on glycemic levels. Diabetic women concurrently treated with β2 adrenoreceptor agonist as a tocolytic drug used to stop or postpone premature labor, needed more insulin than those without this treatment.[30]

As a result of offered evidences and the fact that the prevalence of pregnancies complicated by diabetes is increasing, the need for the answers to unsolved questions regarding use of ACS in preexisting, overt, or gestational diabetes mellitus is present. Regrettably, women with these conditions have been left out from most randomized controlled trials of ACS therapy due to worries about the possible effects on glycemic control.[26] In the systematic review and meta-analysis by Amiya et al., available evidences on ACS use among special subgroups of women at risk of imminent preterm birth were synthesized.[33] The authors acknowledged no eligible studies for ACS use in diabetic pregnant women and concluded that there is no evidence to clearly demonstrate the benefits or harms of ACS in this population of women.[33] However, they found indirect confirmations that advocate the precaution in use of ACS in such patients.[33]

Notwithstanding of presented facts, clinical guideline proclaimed by the National Institute for Health and Clinical Excellence states "diabetes should not be considered a contraindication to ACS".[34] The standard antenatal corticosteroid pattern can be used in diabetes. However, the choice of ACS should be customized for each patient individually, based on the benefit to risk ratio in specific clinical situation and availability of neonatal care. In making the decision in uncertain cases, judgment should be done in a team made by obstetrician, neonatologist and endocrinologist. We must be aware that in severely ill pregnant women with diabetic ketoacidosis or in pregnancies complicated with diabetes together with fulminant infection, ACS treatment must be avoided because it may put at risk maternal health, which should take priority over fetal prophylaxis.[35]

In the Roberts CPG version 2015 systematic review of single course of ACS in women at risk of preterm birth, 5 of 26 trials in total have been reported with study population which encompassed subpopulation of participants who had diabetes.[26] The percentage of women enrolled with pregnancy complicated with diabetes was in range from 2% to 18%. A significant increase of maternal glycemic levels was found only in one trial of women with severe preeclampsia. On the other hand, no significant differences were found in postnatal pyrexia, puerperal sepsis and chorioamnionitis between pregnant women with diabetes and other subpopulations of pregnant participants. Observed neonatal outcomes were perinatal death, neonatal death and neonatal RDS and no significant differences were found between pregnant women with diabetes and other subpopulations of pregnant participants. Since these evidences were established only from a subset of data from trials that included a proportion of women with diabetes in pregnancy, further randomized trials of ACS have to assess the effect on maternal glucose tolerance. Furthermore, this level of evidence cannot be used to form clinical recommendation. However, some good practice points based on the clinical experience of the several guideline development groups are:[36,37]

- The existence of maternal diabetes in pregnancy is not a reason to hold back ACS where there is a risk of preterm birth.
- These women will necessitate blood glucose checking and management of hyperglycemia in accordance with local protocols.

Repeated antenatal corticosteroid prophylaxis was analyzed in the Crowther Cochrane systematic review.[38] Amongst 10 analyzed clinical trials, there were 4 reported participants with diabetes in pregnancy. However, the proportion of those women was small, ranging from 5% to 10%. Repeated ACS did not have significantly different outcomes regarding the risk for chorioamnionitis, puerperal sepsis, perinatal, fetal and neonatal death among those with repeated ACS and those with no repeated treatment. Furthermore, those women with pregnancies complicated with diabetes did not have significantly different outcomes compared to other pregnant women. The data on risk for RDS after repeated ACS demonstrated significantly decreased risk compared to women with no repeat exposure to ACS. Trials that included subpopulation of pregnant women with diabetes have shown that the magnitude of the treatment result in this subgroup was comparable to the overall effect and no significant differences have been found. Observed neonatal outcomes were perinatal death, neonatal death and neonatal RDS and no significant differences were found between pregnant women with diabetes and other subpopulations of pregnant participants. Since these data were obtained only from a subcategory of records from trials that involved a proportion of women with pregnancy complicated with diabetes, additional randomized trials of ACS should evaluate the effect on maternal glucose tolerance. Besides, this level of evidence cannot be used to form clinical endorsement. However, there are some practice points recommended by experts of several renowned medical societies such as:[36,37]

- Maternal diabetes in pregnancy does not justify avoidance of ACS use in women with a risk of preterm birth.
- These women will necessitate blood glucose monitoring and management of hyperglycemia as per local protocols.

## RECOMMENDATIONS FOR MANAGEMENT POLICY FOR WOMEN WITH PREEXISTING DIABETES REQUIRING ANTENATAL CORTICOSTEROID THERAPY

Indications for ACS in this subpopulation of pregnant women are imminent preterm delivery before 36 weeks of gestation, elective cesarean delivery before 39 weeks of pregnancy and planned delivery prior to 36 weeks of gestation due to maternal and/or fetal reasons.[36,37] As mentioned previously, personalized plan should be made for each patient. In order to postpone the labor, β2 adrenoreceptor agonist as a tocolytic drug must be avoided and atosiban should be used.[30] It is mandatory to report to neonatal unit about the presence of such patient.

The betamethasone administrated at two doses intramuscularly 12 hours apart is recommended for pregnant women with preexisting diabetes. Insulin sliding scale should be applied after ACS injection.[37] Infusion of insulin should consists of 50 units of human Actrapid insulin in 50 mL of normal saline solution in a 50 mL syringe (1 mL of insulin solution contains 1 unit of insulin). Application of insulin should be done with syringe pump because the rate of infusion should be determined by the sliding scale (Table 8.1). It is important to give insulin and dextrose via the same cannula using a Y connector. Glucose infusion should be made from 5% solution of dextrose with 20 mmol potassium chloride and should be given by using Gemini pump. Hourly monitoring of glycemic levels should be performed in patients who

| Table 8.1: The sliding scale for determination of insulin infusion rate. | | | | | | |
|---|---|---|---|---|---|---|
| Blood glucose levels | <4.0 | 4.1–6.0 | 6.1–9.0 | 9.1–12.0 | 12.1–15.0 | >15.0 |
| Insulin infusion rate | 0.5*# | 1.0 | 2.0 | 3.0 | 4.0 | 6.0 |

*Stop insulin infusion for 15 minutes and treat hypoglycemia orally with glucogel or with 50 mL of 20% solution of dextrose
#Insulin rate of 0 mL/hour can be maintained if blood glucose is less than 4 mmol in women with type 2 diabetes.

do not mandate adjustment of the insulin rate.[37] However, in patients whose blood glucose levels are requiring the alteration of the insulin rate, glycemia should be checked at every 30 minutes.[37]

One of the goals of this protocol is to keep glucose levels in the range of 4–7 mmol/L prior and during the labor in order to decrease the risk of neonatal hypoglycemia.[37] Another important aim is to maintain the wellbeing of pregnant women and mother. Therefore, if blood glucose level is above 10 mmol/L or if patient is not feeling well it is obligatory to check for ketonuria presence. It is important to look for advice from diabetic team if blood glucose levels in women on sliding scale are not retained below 8 mmol/L. Furthermore, insulin infusion rate should be halved on delivery of placenta to avoid risk of hypoglycemia and insulin infusion should be continued until the patient is ready to eat and drink.[37]

## RECOMMENDATIONS FOR MANAGEMENT POLICY FOR WOMEN WITH GESTATIONAL DIABETES REQUIRING ANTENATAL CORTICOSTEROID THERAPY

The use of ACS is intended for women with imminent or emerging preterm birth before 36 gestational weeks, planned delivery before 36 gestational weeks due to fetal or maternal reasons and for those patients undergoing elective cesarean section before 39 weeks of gestation.[36,37] The betamethasone administrated at two doses intramuscularly 12 hours apart is recommended for pregnant women with gestational diabetes. Management of women with gestational diabetes should be tailor-made according to the class of gestational diabetes. Women with class A2 gestational diabetes requiring insulin should be admitted to clinic and after the first dose of ACS sliding scale should take place and be finished 24 hours after the second dose of ACS.[37] Women with class A1 gestational diabetes, both those who are on metformin or on diet, are discharged from clinic after the administration of ACS.[37] However, they are monitored for blood glucose levels pre- and postmeal in clinic and are obliged to check glycemic levels 7 times a day at home (pre and post meal levels and bed-time level). Those who have one level above 10 mmol/L or two readings higher than 8 mmol/L should refer for sliding scale.[37] Sliding scale in women with gestational diabetes should be discontinued after delivery of placenta. First 48 hours preprandial blood glucose levels (before breakfast, lunch and dinner) should be undertaken.

## RECOMMENDATIONS FOR MANAGEMENT POLICY FOR WOMEN WITH DIABETES REQUIRING ANTENATAL CORTICOSTEROID THERAPY IN THE SETTING WITH PREDOMINATELY SUBCUTANEOUS INSULIN TREATMENT

In attempts to tighten glycemic control after ACS use in pregnant women with imminent premature birth and diabetes, several authors established specific procedures of insulin dosage. Mathiesen et al. developed an algorithm for improved subcutaneous insulin treatment during glucocorticoid treatment in insulin-dependent diabetic women in order to avoid poor glycemic control.[39] This algorithm endorses the increase of insulin dose of 40% shortly after glucocorticoid treatment for fetal lung maturation in diabetic women.

Alternatively, Kaushal et al. proposed a protocol for improved glycemic control following corticosteroid therapy in diabetic pregnant women on subcutaneous insulin treatment.[40] Subcutaneous insulin and diet are continued, but from the first dexamethasone dose until 12 hours after the second, supplementary intravenous insulin is infused according to hourly blood glucose measurements. The protocol incorporates four-graded sliding scales. The initial scale is selected according to the patient's current subcutaneous insulin dose and advanced if the blood glucose is more than or equal to 10.1 mmol/L for two consecutive hours.[40]

## CONTEMPORARY TESTING OF FETAL LUNG MATURITY IN PREDICTING THE RISK OF RESPIRATORY DISTRESS SYNDROME IN PREGNANCIES COMPLICATED WITH DIABETES BY MAGNETIC RESONANCE IMAGING

Evaluation of fetal lung maturity is of great help in predicting the risk of RDS in neonate and relies on surfactant-related lipid concentrations in amniotic fluid. Such testing may provide valuable information regarding the need for ACS prophylaxis of RDS but it is required to collect specimens during amniocentesis. Invasive antenatal testing, such as amniocentesis, carries risks for the fetus and mother, although these risks are very low. ACS given for acceleration of fetal lung maturation significantly increase lung to liver signal-intensity ratios on magnetic resonance imaging. This increase most likely reveals altering properties of the fetal lung parenchyma.[41] Therefore, magnetic resonance, as harmless and noninvasive diagnostic tool, should be considered in evaluation of fetal lung maturity in high risk pregnancies (such as those complicated with diabetes) instead of biochemical testing enabled by invasive and risk carrying amniocentesis.

## CONTEMPORARY ROLE OF ULTRASONOGRAPHY IN PREGNANCIES COMPLICATED WITH DIABETES WITH EMPHASIS ON THOSE THAT REQUIRE ANTENATAL STEROID THERAPY

Ultrasonography is noninvasive, readily available diagnostic procedure with high acceptance and compliance among obstetric patients. Wide acceptance of ultrasonography, alongside with its technology breakthroughs, allows the spreading out the use of ultrasound in those screening, diagnostic and therapeutic fields in which ultrasonography was neither present nor conceivable in the past. Such new roles of ultrasound in pregnancies complicated with diabetes are those related to ultrasound based:

- Screening for gestational diabetes
- Estimation of fetal weight
- Management of therapy
- Evaluation of fetal lung maturity.

Numerous studies have demonstrated high diagnostic performances of ultrasound findings in detection of gestational diabetes, both from usual screening period and onwards (from 24th to 36th weeks of gestation)[42-44] and before usual screening period.[45,46] This kind of detection of gestational diabetes was based either on measurement and evaluation of only one ultrasound marker of gestational diabetes, such as fetal subcutaneous fat tissue[44] or fetal liver,[45] etc. or on measurement and evaluation of multiple ultrasound markers[43,46] or even with performing the ultrasound score for detection of gestational diabetes by using nine ultrasound markers of gestational diabetes.[42] Therefore, ultrasound has been recognized as modern supplementary screening tool for gestational diabetes. Furthermore, the role of ultrasound examinations is well established in estimation of fetal weight, in diagnosis of congenital malformation and in monitoring diabetic pregnant patients.[47]

Taking into account wide acceptance and compliance of obstetric ultrasound examinations and the high rate of administration of unnecessarily ACS,[48] new diagnostic approach in ultrasound evaluation of fetal lung maturity has been established.[49] Some elusive changes in the characteristic or texture of ultrasound images invisible to the human eye could be ascertained by computerized methods of texture analysis of medical images.[50] These powerful computerized quantitative methods for ultrasound image analysis were developed due to progresses in computer capacity and image resolution. As a result, these textural arrangements were used to train algorithms to envisage clinical information.

Serizawa and Maeda put out a form of tissue characterization known as ultrasonic gray-level histogram width, which combined with gestational age, anticipated the occurrence of RDS.[51] The diagnostic performances of the method were as good as with invasive amniotic fluid tests, with sensitivity and specificity of 0.96 and 0.72, respectively. The main clinical limitation of the method was the fact that it requires analysis of multiple fetal organs, the lung and the liver. On the other hand, the major methodological constraint was reduced sample of participant (22 and 25 fetuses with and without RDS in turn). Nevertheless, the study outcomes were encouraging.[51]

Texture evaluation of fetal lung ultrasound images is capable to fathom patterns of features that strongly correlate with gestational age,[52] or with the results of fetal lung maturity tests on amniotic fluid.[53] Demonstrated correlations and associations were not influenced by delineation parameters such as region of interest localization and size, right to left lung selected or ultrasonographic parameters, for instance, used transducer or type of ultrasound equipment which is important for widespread use of the method.[52] Aforementioned studies delivered a proof of concept of the prospective of texture-based approaches, but common difficulties of other quantitative imaging methods remained, for instance the absence of validity of blind testing due to variable acquisition conditions. For that reason, Bonet-Carne et al. tested the ability of texture analysis of fetal lung ultrasound images to predict blindly the risk of neonatal respiratory morbidity and to address aforementioned limitations by developing a new method, called termed "quantitative ultrasound fetal lung maturity analysis" (quantusFLM™), which combines various image texture extractors and machine learning algorithms.[49] Firstly, they used more than 13,000 nonclinical images and 900 fetal lung images to develop a method based on texture analysis and machine learning algorithms, trained to predict neonatal respiratory morbidity risk on fetal lung ultrasound images. QuantusFLM™ was subsequently confirmed blindly in 144 neonates, delivered at 28+0 to 39+0 weeks' gestation. Lung ultrasound images in Digital Imaging and Communications in Medicine (DICOM) format were acquired within 48 hours of delivery and the capability of the software to predict neonatal respiratory morbidity, defined as either RDS or transient tachypnea of the newborn, was determined. There were

29 (20.1%) cases of neonatal respiratory morbidity among neonates. Quantitative texture analysis predicted neonatal respiratory morbidity with a sensitivity, specificity, positive predictive value and negative predictive value of 86.2%, 87.0%, 62.5% and 96.2%, respectively. Since the quantitative ultrasound fetal lung maturity analysis predicted neonatal respiratory morbidity with accuracy equivalent to that of current tests using amniotic fluid, this method can significantly reduce unnecessarily antenatal steroid therapy by refining the decision to whom ACS should be given.

## REFERENCES

1. Liggins GC. The role of cortisol in preparing the fetus for birth. Reprod Fertil Dev. 1994;6(2):141-50.
2. Blencowe H, Cousens S, Oestergaard M, et al. National, regional and worldwide estimates of preterm birth. Lancet. 2012;379(9832):2162-72.
3. Rossi S. Corticosteroids. In: Rossi S (Ed). Australian Medicines Handbook, 7th illustrated edition. Adelaide: Australian Medicines Handbook; 2006. pp. 496-500.
4. Ballard PL, Ballard RA. Scientific basis and therapeutic regiments for use of antenatal glucocorticoids. Am J Obstet Gynecol. 1995;173:254-62.
5. Gnanalingham MG, Mostyn A, Gardner DS, et al. Developmental regulation of the lung in preparation for life after birth: hormonal and nutritional manipulation of local glucocorticoid action and uncoupling protein-2. J Endocrinol. 2006;188(3):375-86.
6. Ikegami M, Polk DH, Jobe AH, et al. Effect of interval from fetal corticosteroid treatment to delivery on postnatal lung function of preterm lambs. J Appl Physiol (1985). 1996;80(2):591-7.
7. Ballard PL, Ertsey R, Gonzales W, et al. Transcriptional regulation of human pulmonary surfactant proteins SP-B and SP-C by glucocorticoids. Am J Respir Cell Mol Biol. 1996;14:599-607.
8. NIH Consensus Development panel on the effect of corticosteroids for fetal maturation on perinatal outcomes. Effect of corticosteroids for fetal maturation on perinatal outcomes. JAMA. 1995;273(5):413-8.
9. Berger PJ, Smolich JJ, Ramsden CA, et al. Effect of lung liquid volume on respiratory performance after caesarean delivery in the lamb. J Physiol. 1996;492:905-12.
10. Irestedt L, Lagercrantz H, Belfrage P. Causes and consequences of maternal and fetal symapaticoadrenal activation during parturition. Acta Obstet Gynecol Scand. 1984;Suppl 181:111-5.
11. Riley CA, Boozer K, King TL. Antenatal corticosteroids at the beginning of the 21st century. J Midwifery Womens Health. 2011;56:591-7.
12. Jain L, Eaton DC. Physiology of fetal lung fluid clearance and the effect of labor. Semin Perinatol. 2006;30:34-43.
13. Moore TR. A comparison of amniotic fluid fetal pulmonary phospholipids in normal and diabetic pregnancy. Am J Obstet Gynecol. 2002;186(4):641-50.
14. Piper JM, Xenakis EM, Langer O. Delayed appearance of pulmonary maturation markers is associated with poor glucose control in diabetic pregnancies. J Matern Fetal Med. 1998;7(3):148-53.
15. Treviño-Alanís M, Ventura-Juárez J, Hernández-Piñero J, et al. Delayed lung maturation of foetus of diabetic mother rats develop with a diminish, but without changes in the proportion of type I and II pneumocytes, and decreased expression of protein D-associated surfactant factor. Anat Histol Embryol. 2009;38(3):169-76.
16. Tegethoff M, Pryce C, Meinschmidt G. Effects of intrauterine exposure to synthetic glucocorticoids on fetal, newborn, and infant hypothalamic-pituitary-adrenal axis function in humans: a systematic review. Endocr Rev. 2009;30:753-89.
17. Liggins GC. Premature delivery of foetal lambs infused with glucocorticoids. J Endocrinol. 1969;45(4):515-23.
18. Liggins GC, Howie RN. A controlled trial of antepartum glucocorticoid treatment for prevention of respiratory distress syndrome in premature infants. Pediatrics. 1972;50(4):515-25.

19. Crowley P. Prophylactic corticosteroids for preterm birth. Cochrane Database Syst Rev. 2002;(2):CD000065.
20. NIH Consensus Development Conference statement. Effect of corticosteroids for fetal maturation on perinatal outcomes. NIH Consensus Statement. 1994;12(2):1-24.
21. Crowley PA. Antenatal corticosteroid therapy: a meta-analysis of the randomized trials, 1972 to 1994. Am J Obstet Gynecol. 1995;173:322-35.
22. Baud O, Foix-L'Helias L, Kaminski M, et al. Antenatal glucocorticoid treatment and cystic periventricular leukomalacia in very premature infants. N Engl J Med. 1999;341:1190-6.
23. Robert MF, Neff RK, Hubbell JP, et al. Association between maternal diabetes and respiratory distress syndrome in the newborn. N Engl J Med. 1976;294:357-60.
24. Royal College of Obstetricians and Gynaecologists (RCOG). Antenatal corticosteroids to prevent respiratory distress syndrome. Clinical Green Top Guidelines. Royal College of Obstetricians and Gynaecologists, 2004.
25. Committee Opinion No. 677. ACOG committee opinion: antenatal corticosteroids therapy for fetal maturation. Obstet Gynecol. 2016;128:e187-94.
26. Roberts D, Dalziel S. Antenatal corticosteroids for accelerating fetal lung maturation for women at risk of preterm birth. Cochrane Database Syst Rev. 2006;19:CD004454.
27. Saccone G, Berghella V. Antenatal corticosteroids for maturity of term or near term fetuses:systematic review and meta-analysis of randomized controlled trials. BMJ. 2016;355:i5044.
28. Sibai BM, Caritis SN, Hauth JC, et al. Preterm delivery in women with pregestational diabetes or chronic hypertension relative to women with uncomplicated pregnancies. The National Institute of Child Health and Human Development Maternal- Fetal Medicine Units Network. Am J Obstet Gynecol. 2000;183(6):1520-4.
29. JianYun X, Zhaoxia L, Yun C, et al. Changes in maternal glucose metabolism after the administration of dexamethasone for fetal lung development. Int J Endocrinol Metab. 2012;2012:652806.
30. Refuerzo JS, Garg A, Rech B, et al. Continuous glucose monitoring in diabetic women following antenatal corticosteroid therapy: a pilot study. Am J Perinatol. 2012;29(5):335-8.
31. Itoh A, Saisho Y, Miyakoshi K, et al. Time-dependent changes in insulin requirement for maternal glycemic control during antenatal corticosteroid therapy in women with gestational diabetes: a retrospective study. Endocr J. 2016;63(1):101-4.
32. Jolley JA, Rajan PV, Petersen R, et al. Effect of antenatal betamethasone on blood glucose levels in women with and without diabetes. Diabetes Res Clin Pract. 2016;118:98-104.
33. Amiya RM, Mlunde LB, Ota E, et al. Antenatal corticosteroids for reducing adverse maternal and child outcomes in special populations of women at risk of imminent preterm birth: a systematic review and meta-analysis. PLoS One. 2016;11(2):e0147604.
34. National Institute of Health and Clinical Excellence. Diabetes in pregnancy: Management of diabetes and its complications from preconception to the postnatal period. 2015. [online] NICE Guideline 2015. Available from: https://www.nice.org.uk/guidance/ng3/resources/diabetes-in-pregnancy-management-of-diabetes-and-its-complications-from-preconception-to-the-postnatal-period-51038446021. [Accessed August 2017].
35. Kalra S, Kalra B, Gupta Y. Glycemic management after antenatal corticosteroid therapy. N Am J Med Sci. 2014;6(2):71-6.
36. Royal College of Obstetricians and Gynaecologists. Antenatal corticosteroids to reduce neonatal morbidity and mortality. Green–top Guideline No. 7. 2010. [online] Available from: https://www.rcog.org.uk/globalassets/documents/guidelines/gtg_7.pdf [Accessed August 2017].
37. Antenatal Corticosteroid Clinical Practice Guidelines Panel. Antenatal corticosteroids given to women prior to birth to improve fetal, infant, child and adult health: Clinical Practice Guidelines. Liggins Institute, the University of Auckland, Auckland; 2015. New Zealand.
38. Crowther CA, McKinlay CJ, Middleton P, et al. Repeat doses of prenatal corticosteroids for women at risk of preterm birth for improving neonatal health outcomes. Cochrane Database Syst Rev. 2011;(6):CD003935.

39. Mathiesen ER, Christensen AB, Hellmuth E, et al. Insulin dose during glucocorticoid treatment for fetal lung maturation in diabetic pregnancy: test of an algorithm [correction of algorithm]. Acta Obstet Gynecol Scand. 2002;81(9):835-9.

40. Kaushal K, Gibson JM, Railton A, et al. A protocol for improved glycemic control following cortico-steroid therapy in diabetic pregnancies. Diabet Med. 2003;20(1):73-5.

41. Schmid M, Kasprian G, Kuessel L, et al. Effect of antenatal corticosteroid treatment on the fetal lung: a magnetic resonance imaging study. Ultrasound Obstet Gynecol. 2011;38:94-8.

42. Perović M, Garalejić E, Gojnić M, et al. Sensitivity and specificity of ultrasonography as a screening tool for gestational diabetes mellitus. J Matern Fetal Neonatal Med. 2012;25 (8):1348-53.

43. Gojnić M, Stefanović T, Perović M, et al. Prediction of fetal macrosomia with ultrasound para-meters and maternal glycemic controls in gestational diabetes mellitus. Clin Exp Obstet Gynecol. 2013;39(4):512-5.

44. Tantanasis T, Daniilidis A, Giannoulis C, et al. Sonographic assessment of fetal subcutaneous fat tissue thickness as an indicator of gestational diabetes. Eur J Obstet Gynecol Reprod Biol. 2010;152(2):157-62.

45. Perovic M, Gojnic M, Arsic B, et al. Relationship between mid-trimester ultrasound fetal liver length measurements and gestational diabetes mellitus. J Diabetes. 2015;7(4):497-505.

46. Mirghani H, Zayed R, Thomas L, et al. Gestational diabetes mellitus: fetal liver length measure-ments between 21 and 24 weeks' gestation. J Clin Ultrasound. 2007;35(1):34-7.

47. Ahmed B, Abushama M, Khraisheh M, et al. Role of ultrasound in the management of diabetes in pregnancy. J Matern Fetal Neonatal Med. 2015;28(15):1856-63.

48. Sanya R, Al Naggar E, Gasim M, et al. Use or overuse of antenatal corticosteroids for suspected preterm birth. J Matern Fetal Neonatal Med. 2014;27(14):1454-6.

49. Bonet-Carne E, Palacio M, Cobo T, et al. Quantitative ultrasound texture analysis of fetal lungs to predict neonatal respiratory morbidity. Ultrasound Obstet Gynecol. 2015;45(4):427-33.

50. Bergen JR, Adelson E. Theories of visual texture perception. Spat Vis. 1991;10:114-34.

51. Serizawa M, Maeda K. Noninvasive fetal lung maturity prediction based on ultrasonic gray level histogram width. Ultrasound Med Biol. 2010;36:1998-2003.

52. Cobo T, Bonet-Carne E, Martınez-Terron M, et al. Feasibility and reproducibility of fetal lung texture analysis by automatic quantitative ultrasound analysis and correlation with gestational age. Fetal Diagn Ther. 2012;31:230-6.

53. Palacio M, Cobo T, Martınez-Terron M, et al. Performance of an automatic quantitative ultrasound analysis of the fetal lung to predict fetal lung maturity. Am J Obstet Gynecol. 2012;207:504.e1-5.

# Chapter 9

# Diabetes and Obesity in Pregnancy

*Hisham Arab*

## INTRODUCTION

The global obesity epidemic has resulted in heavier women in the reproductive age. More than 30% of women are above the ideal weight at the onset of their pregnancy. Similarly, there are more obese women suffering from type I or type II diabetes mellitus (DM).[1] The risk of gestational diabetes mellitus (GDM) is strongly linked to increasing maternal body mass index (BMI). This statement has been reiterated in all publications regardless of its location, study design and analytical method for the past 25 years. The best representative study of all is a meta-analysis that reviewed 20 studies published over a period of 15 years and reported the unadjusted odds ratio of developing GDM was 2.14 in overweight women, while that for obese, and severely obese women were 3.56 and 8.56, respectively, when compared with normal weight pregnant women.[2] In the absence of DM, obesity alone is also considered an obstetric risk factor. Maternal and fetal outcome and corrective measures of this complex triad is the subject of this chapter.

## BURDEN OF A DISEASE: INFLUENCING MATERNAL MORTALITY RATE

World Health Organization (WHO) announced lately that worldwide obesity has more than doubled since 1980. In their 2014 report, they calculated that 15% of adult women (above the age of 18 years) were obese, while additional 40% were overweight. In Mexico, the incidence is nearly doubled; 70% of women are overweight and almost half of them are obese.[3] As a result their 2016 maternal mortality rate (MMR) report was astonishing.[4]

Maternal mortality rate is now classified into two cause-dependent categories: (1) direct (obstetrically related) and (2) indirect (maternal deaths resulted from preexisting disease that worsen by pregnancy). The latter includes pregnancies complicated by DM, cardiovascular, infectious, and other diseases. Data from this 8-year study period from Mexico indicated that direct MMR had declined from 46.4 to 32.1 per 100,000 live births while indirect MMR had slightly risen from 12.2 to 13.3 deaths per 100,000 live births. This study supports the newly witnessed shift in the causes of maternal deaths from direct to indirect; a phenomenon that has been referred to lately as the "obstetric transition". Socioeconomic status plays a great role in this transition as the number of better-educated and wealthier women who suffer from obesity and high levels of cholesterol are on the rise in recent years.[5] The impact of obesity per se on mortality in general is well-documented. A number of large-scale prospective studies have shown that the risk of death is highly associated with lower and higher BMI categories than the middle BMI range.[6]

## Do Women See Themselves Overweight?

The WHO classification of adult weight according to BMI was published in 1995 and updated few times since then.[7] Table 9.1 depicts an adaptation from such publications. Both overweight and normal-weight women commonly misperceive their body weight. A study from North Carolina University was presented at the 2006 congress on Experimental Biology reported that only 15% of women meeting the obesity criteria of the National Institutes of Health realized they were obese. In another study, however, 25% of women felt the same, while 17% of normal weight women misperceived themselves as overweight.[8] More recently, the latter group conducted a survey on obesity risk knowledge, dieting, and weight misperception among women planning to become pregnant and found that 31% misperceived their body weight, 51% had little knowledge about the risk of obesity, and 76% had poor knowledge of healthy diet. Weight misperception was more pronounced among overweight than obese women intending to become pregnant (71% vs 10%; P < 0.001).[9]

## OBESITY AND GESTATIONAL DIABETES MELLITUS: ARE THEY INDEPENDENT?

While the prevalence of obesity in reproductive age is 63%,[10] more than 50% of pregnant women are either overweight or obese.[11] On the other hand, GDM affects 1–14% of all pregnancies depending on the genetic and environmental factors as well as screening and diagnostic methods employed in various sources.[12] Its prevalence can even be as high as 18% in a country like Saudi Arabia, which is one of the highest regions and the world.[13] There is no doubt that either obesity or GDM has adverse pregnancy outcome, but it is worse when both conditions coexist.[14] The independent effect of maternal BMI and maternal hyperglycemia on the pregnancy outcome, however, has only been investigated in few studies. One of them showed a greater independent effect of obesity on adverse pregnancy outcomes, such as macrosomia, cesarean delivery, and pregnancy-induced hypertension, compared to GDM.[15] Although independent association with adverse pregnancy outcomes of maternal obesity and GDM was also shown in a recent retrospective cohort study; their findings confirmed that the

**Table 9.1:** WHO classification of adult weight according to BMI.

| Underweight—Normal range | BMI | Overweight—Obese | BMI |
|---|---|---|---|
| Underweight | <18.5 | Overweight | ≥ 25.0 |
| Severe thinness | <16.0 | Preobese | 25.0–29.9 |
| Moderate thinness | 16.0–16.9 | Obese | ≥ 30.0 |
| Mild thinness | 17.0–18.5 | Class I | 30.0–34.9 |
| | | Class II | 35.0–39.9 |
| Normal weight | 18.5–24.9 | Class III | ≥ 40.0 |

(BMI: Body mass index; WHO: World Health Organization)

combination of both GDM and obesity had greater impact on macrosomia and CS delivery than either GDM or obesity alone.[16] Other investigators have specifically reported a greater impact of maternal obesity on the adverse pregnancy outcomes than that of GDM.[17]

## OBESITY AND GESTATIONAL DIABETES MELLITUS: FUTURE RISK

A woman's weight at the onset of pregnancy is the best predictor of her child's future health and weight status. Gene modulation during the antenatal period constitutes an epigenetic effect on the embryo that is specific for each individual pregnancy. Maternal weight and its biological consequences at the onset of pregnancy make that distinct effect. This is why children born to the same mother have different risks depending on her prepregnancy weight.

The second detrimental factor of a child's risk of developing obesity is maternal weight gain over the course of pregnancy. It is a good practice to follow the maternal weight gain guidelines published by the American Institute of Medicine in 2009 (Table 9.2). Excessive maternal weight gain in obese and GDM women is associated with increased insulin resistance (IR) that leads to a trail of events starting with fetal macrosomia and future increased incidence of obesity and glucose intolerance in their offspring.[18] Obviously, genetic factors may explain the dietary and physical behavior similarities between mother and offspring which may contribute to this association;[19] furthermore, type 2 diabetes rates in future generations could also increase as a causal effect possibility. The pregnancy weight gain of overweight and obese Swedish mothers was found to correlate very well with their sons BMI at the age of 18 years, as shown in a large study on 150,000 Swedish army recruits. This correlation was not found in normal weight mothers. This further strengthens the significance of weight gain during pregnancy and its impact on future risk on offspring.

In addition, there are sporadic publications linking obesity/GDM with childhood complications such as childhood cancer, autism, asthma, and cardiomyopathy. Such findings need further research and replication from other sources.

## OBESITY AND GESTATIONAL DIABETES MELLITUS: ADVERSE PREGNANCY OUTCOME

Obese mothers always carry the risk of developing GDM, preeclampsia, hypertension, or undergo labor induction or primary CS with increased likelihood of preterm births and stillbirths.

**Table 9.2:** Recommended weight gains in pregnancy according to prepregnancy BMI.

| BMI at onset of pregnancy | Targeted total weight gain (kg) | Approximate weekly weight gain (kg/week) from the 15th week |
|---|---|---|
| Underweight <18.5 | 12–18 | 0.5 |
| Normal weight 18.5–24.9 | 11–15 | 0.5 |
| Overweight 25.0–29.9 | 7–11 | 0.3 |
| Obese (all classes) ≥30.0 | 5–9 | 0.2 |

(BMI: Body mass index)

Likewise, complications related to excessive weight gain during pregnancy and macrosomia include emergency CS, shoulder dystocia, clavicle fractures, brachial plexus injury, depressed 5-minute Apgar scores and increased rates of admission to neonatal intensive care unit;[20] as well as maternal physical injury and postpartum hemorrhage.[21]

## Congenital Anomalies

It is well established that GDM does not cause congenital malformation; it is only preexisting uncontrolled DM that is highly associated with cardiac and neural tube defects (NTD). The story is different for obese women.

Compared with normal weight women, obese and severely obese women have two- and threefold risk of NTD, respectively.[22] This could be attributed to lack of nutritional supplements as women with a BMI greater than or equal to 27 are less likely to use them and consequently suffer from folate deficiency.[23] Accordingly, women with higher BMI should receive higher doses of folate supplementation in order to reduce risk of fetal NTDs.

## Fetal Macrosomia

We have known for years the Pedersen hypothesis[24] that explains the pathophysiology of fetal macrosomia in women with GDM. It simply describes how the facilitated diffusion of glucose across the placenta mirrors the maternal hyperglycemia in fetal circulation resulting in fetal hyperinsulinemia; which is evidenced recently by high insulin levels in the cord blood of babies born to diabetic mothers.[25] As a result, both fetal glucose utilization and fat deposition in GDM are increased.

Through a genetic link the parents' weight and height may influence fetal weight. Maternal weight can modulate the intrauterine environment through its biochemical milieu of hyperinsulinemia, hyperlipidemia and increased inflammatory markers levels.[26,27] More precisely, fetal size correlates with the level of circulating maternal lipids in the 3rd trimester rather than glucose level.[28,29] Hence, macrosomia is more commonly associated with maternal obesity or both obesity and GDM rather than GDM alone. Diagrammatic representation of this complex issue of fetal macrosomia is shown in Figure 9.1.

This is why we still see macrosomic fetuses in well-controlled GDM patients, which means other obesity-related mediators might play a significant role in the establishment of macrosomia.[30]

Smith and his group from UK[31] noted that by the time clinical diagnosis of GDM was established at 28 weeks gestation excessive fetal growth has already started. In such patients, there is increased growth velocity between 20 weeks and 28 weeks resulting in threefold increased risk of AC or HC/AC above 90 the centile at 28 weeks and macrosomia at birth. Accordingly, in order to improve the short- and long-term outcomes of pregnancies complicated by GDM early universal screening should be practiced despite the current recommendation of biochemical testing for GDM between 24 weeks and 28 weeks adopted by major organizations like the American College of Obstetricians and Gynecologists (ACOG) and the National Institute For Health and Clinical Excellence (NICE).

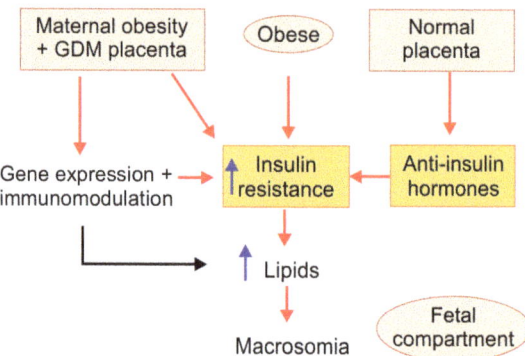

**Fig. 9.1:** Multifactorial representation of possible causes of fetal macrosomia.

## Cesarean Section Rate

When compared to normal weight women, obese women are at two- to threefold increased risk of CS.[32] After adjustment for comorbidity like GDM, Dietz et al. reported similar findings.[33] Wahabi and her group from Saudi Arabia also found that this risk is independently associated with obesity and that GDM has not inflicted extra risk for CS delivery over that anticipated from maternal obesity. Possible reasons that explain the association between obesity and high CS rate include cephalopelvic disproportion,[34] failure to progress in labor[35] and higher labor emergencies such as abnormal cardiotocographic tracing.[36]. Finally, it is worth mentioning that there are certain CS complications which are seen mostly in obese women such as venous thromboembolism, extended hospitalization period, urinary tract infection, endomyometritis, and wound infection.[37]

## Preeclampsia

Contrary to lean women, pregnant obese patients tend to have certain degree of high blood pressure, and altered cardiac function with hemoconcentration.[38]

The incidence of hypertension is 2.2–21.4 times higher in obese women than in control subjects, and preeclampsia occurs 1.2–9.7 times more often.[39] During pregnancy, truncal or central obesity remains a risk factor to develop hypertension as in nonpregnant women.[40] Adverse metabolic and vascular effects of overweight and obesity are particularly seen in visceral obesity. Thus, it is not merely the actual BMI, but also fat mass distributions that reflect risk of PET.

Although hypertension in obese women is associated with a reduction in subcutaneous fat of the newborn, the incidence of small-for-gestational-age infants is usually similar to that in normal-weight subjects.

It is well documented that obesity predisposes a woman to preeclampsia whether she is diabetic or not.[41,42] Insulin resistance, subclinical inflammation, and lipotoxicity are common features of both obesity and preeclampsia.[43,44] Lipotoxicity in obese pregnant women causes maternal vascular dysfunction and reduced trophoblast invasion that may explain the development of PET in such women. Moreover, the vascular endothelium is further compromised by the reduced endogenous production of nitric oxide that is commonly seen in obesity.[45]

Regardless of BMI, compared with women without DM, PET was six times higher in women with type 1 DM and 3.5 times higher in women with type II DM.[46] Comparison studies of PET in women with type I and type II diabetes are limited and inconsistent.[47,48] Persson and her group from Sweden[49] attributed the higher incidence of PET in type I than type II DM to differences in risk factors, such as the presence of microangiopathy, duration of the disease, chronic hypertension, and the level of glycemic control. Evidence from placental findings suggests that the burden of pregnancy may affect maternal vascularization differently in these two groups.[50] It has been estimated that type I diabetic patients have a 2.5–5% chance of developing diabetic nephropathy when they get pregnant,[51,52] and consequently preeclampsia.[53] Maternal overweight, however, is considered the only indicator of poor pregnancy outcome in type I diabetic pregnant women with nephropathy while duration of diabetes, level of glycemic control and weight gain in pregnancy are not.[54] The presence of microalbuminuria in such patients increases their PET risk by fourfold.[55] Another PET risk factor to be considered here is elevated $HbA_1C$ in early pregnancy.[56,57]

A recent nationwide study from Denmark demonstrated that women with type II diabetes and overt nephropathy or microalbuminuria had comparable rates of preeclampsia to those of women with type I diabetes.[51] Risk factors for women with type II DM are less well studied.[58] Although diabetes per se is a much stronger risk factor of PET than BMI, attaining a normal prepregnancy weight could reduce the risk of PET in diabetic and nondiabetic women.

## Perinatal Death

Maternal obesity is known to be associated with increased risk of perinatal mortality, including fetal, neonatal and infant deaths. According to the Confidential Enquiry into Maternal and Child Health released from UK in 2005, the incidence of maternal obesity among those who had late fetal loss, stillbirth or neonatal death was 22.9%, 30.4%, and 30.6%, respectively.[59] Similar findings were reported by another study where the risk of perinatal death was two to three times greater for women who were obese at the onset of pregnancy compared with normal weight women.[60]

A meta-analysis study on maternal obesity and infant mortality found a linear relationship between BMI and the odds of having an infant death.[61] Birth asphyxia and other neonatal morbidities have been postulated as possible cause of this relationship.[62] More precisely, this degree of increased risk varies according to the timing of fetal or neonatal loss as given in Table 9.3.[63]

Maternal body habitus in obese women may affect the accuracy of estimating fetal weight by ultrasound or monitoring fetal heart during labor, which may lead to adverse outcome, related to misdiagnosis in such patients. There is also some evidence that women who are overweight or obese are less likely to have a live birth following in vitro fertilization.[64]

**Table 9.3:** Risk of fetal or neonatal death associated with every 5 units rise in BMI of obese and overweight pregnant women.

| Timing of death | Mortality risk associated with every 5 units rise in BMI |
|---|---|
| Miscarriage | 16% |
| Fetal death | 21% |
| Stillbirth | 24% |
| Neonatal death | 15% |
| Postneonatal death | 14% |
| Infant death | 18% |

(BMI: Body mass index)

## Premature Births

The risk of preterm birth in obesity for long has been attributed to associate medical complications that necessitate premature interventions, which lead to premature delivery. For example in the presence of preeclampsia, when compared to nondiabetic, the odds ratio of preterm birth is twice in type 1 DM and five times in type 2 DM. However, a recent study of 1 million births in California, USA has found that regardless of race or ethnicity, all obese primigravida were at very high risk of delivery before 28 weeks of gestation. Earlier gestational ages and highest ranks of obesity in this group were associated with the highest risk. It was found that the most obese primigravida group had six times the risk of normal-weight women to deliver before 23 weeks of gestation. It can be concluded that maternal obesity poses a risk of extreme prematurity and not premature deliveries between 28 weeks and 37 weeks of gestation.[65]

## NUTRITIONAL DEPRIVATION IN PREGNANCY

Pregnancy is not the time to loose weight or practice certain dietary regimen to attain a desired shape or figure. However, it is obvious from the above associated risks with obesity that losing weight before pregnancy and optimal weight gain during pregnancy will be the best approach to avoid such complications. In order to advice for the ideal cut we need to examine the extreme of restriction. Starvation and Fasting are the best two examples of prolonged and limited nutritional deprivation, and both are well studied during pregnancy. The outcome of these studies may help guide our recommendation for dieting and weight control of obese patients during pregnancy.

## Starvation

The sympathetic nervous system is most likely suppressed during starvation, which can directly result in decreased metabolic rate along with energy restriction and indirectly limit the energy expenditure through the stimulation of the adreno-medullary system.[66] Drastic reduction in the amount of amino acids in the amniotic fluid in starvation is well-documented in the literature.[67] However, it is unclear at what degree and point of time deprivation will result in an adverse pregnancy outcome. Starting with fasting, glucose levels usually fall, resulting in a drop in insulin secretion and increased gluconeogenesis through the breakdown of glycogen and increased levels of glucagon and catecholamines. After several hours of fasting, more fatty acids will be released from adipocytes as a result of glycogen depletion and hypoinsulinemia. At this point the source of energy for skeletal and cardiac muscle, liver, kidney, and adipose tissue will be the ketones that are generated from the oxidation of fatty acids. Brain and erythrocytes, however, continue to utilize the available glucose as an energy source.[68]

## Fasting

It is clear now that 16-hours of fasting of a pregnant woman will result in significantly lower glucose levels and significantly higher levels of free fatty acids and β-hydroxybutyrate. This was documented in both obese as well as lean women.[69] Fasting during the holy month of Ramadan for Muslims may pose risks to pregnant women. Several studies have pointed out that such women were at risk of poor weight gain with significant change in leptin level,[70] and higher incidence of hyperemesis gravidarum,[71] and low birth weight due to premature labor as a result of increasing levels of placental corticotrophin-releasing hormone in maternal circulation.[72]

## METABOLISM DURING PREGNANCY

### Endocrine Function of Adipose Tissue

Adipose tissue is an endocrine organ that contributes to obesity through its metabolic malfunction.[73] It plays a major role in modifying major hormones storage, secretion, and conversion. Estrone, for example, is converted to estradiol in peripheral adipose tissue. Similarly, cortisone is converted to cortisol through the enzyme 11-i-hydroxysteroid dehydrogenase type 1 that is usually expressed in adipose tissue. In addition to its powerful endocrine function in regulating glucocorticoids, adipose tissue has an immunological function by secreting a large number of bioactive peptides and cytokines (adipokines). In biological terms, obesity is simply a hyperplasia of an endocrine tissue leading to abnormal metabolic changes (Table 9.4).

### Insulin Resistance of Pregnancy

The carbohydrate metabolic changes of pregnancy include postprandial hyperglycemia, hyperinsulinemia, and mild fasting hypoglycemia. In other words, this is state of physiological peripheral IR, which becomes more pronounced following the ingestion of carbohydrate,

| Table 9.4: Specific enzymatic changes in obese pregnant women. | |
|---|---|
| Enzyme | Mode of change |
| Leptin | Increased |
| Adiponectin | Decreased |
| TNF-α | Increased |
| 11-β-OH-steroid dehydrogenase, Type 1 | Increased |

or even pathological in obese pregnant women and gestational diabetes.[74] The daily fetal consumption of glucose in the 3rd trimester is estimated to be around 20–25 g that can best be maintained through this physiologic IR.[75] It has been noted also that this stage of pregnancy is usually associated with high levels of free fatty acids as a result of decreased insulin ability to suppress lipolysis; a form of IR related to lipid metabolism.[76]

"Accelerated starvation in pregnancy" is a term used to describe the increased risk of ketosis in pregnant women. Protein synthesis increases progressively from the 2nd to 3rd trimester, 15% to 25%, respectively. Accordingly, the concentration of amino acids is higher in the fetus than the mother for the purpose of protein synthesis, with only 10% used for oxidation.[77]

## Effect of Obesity on Metabolism during Pregnancy

In a normal weight pregnant woman lipid metabolism switches from lipogenesis in the 1st trimester to lipolysis in the 3rd trimester. Obese women, on the other hand, always live through the state of lipogenesis including the prepregnancy period, but once they get pregnant their metabolism shifts to lipolysis with profound hyperlipidemia throughout all trimesters of pregnancy. Since insulin role is to suppress lipolysis, this is our evidence that obesity is associated with increased IR in all stages of pregnancy. However, IR can be affected by cytokines and inflammatory mediators that are usually secreted by the adipose stromal cells; while TNF-α increases IR and adiponectin reduces it. The effects of obesity on amino acid metabolism are unknown. However, hyperinsulinemia causing decreased protein synthesis in nonpregnant obese women is well established. Accordingly, restricted fetal growth and impaired anabolic response to pregnancy are reasonable assumptions.

## INTERVENTION DURING PREGNANCY

## Safe Weight Loss

Contrary to the common myth "Eat for two", pregnant women do not need additional food throughout their pregnancy. Several studies have shown that well-nourished women with normal pregnancy progression and outcome did not require additional energy intake during pregnancy. The question is where did that all extra energy deposited in new tissues during pregnancy come from? Possible explanations are decline in physical activity or an increase in nutrients absorption. World researchers on this subject have reached a very important and simple consensus that diet and physical activity interventions were effective in reducing pregnancy weight gain.

Energy and protein restricted diet has been tried in pregnant women with overweight, obesity or high gestational weight gain. The results, however, were inconsistent. In obese pregnant women with gestational diabetes, not only 1,200-calorie diet restriction resulted in a better euglycemia but also a significant increase in ketonemia and ketonuria.[78] Contrary to normal diet with low fat and high carbohydrate portions, ketogenic diet consists of high fat and low carbohydrate percentages. Ketogenic diet causes metabolic shift from glycolysis to ketosis. Animal studies have reported that ketones accumulation in fetal compartment as a result of such diet has resulted in variable organ growth with multiple organ dysfunction and possible behavioral deviations in postnatal life.[79] As far as fetal health is concerned, hyperketonemia can

> **Box 9.1:** Ketosis and pregnancy.
>
> - Ketosis is normal during fasting
> - Ketosis implies activation of lipid energy metabolism
> - Ketosis means that the entire pathway of lipolysis is intact
> - Ketosis represents the only nonglucose-derived energy source in the brain
> - Ketosis can be prevented using 1,600–1,700 kcal/day diet as long as 50% of the calories are provided by carbohydrate. Protein and micronutrients are also essential
> - Fetal ketosis as a result of ketogenic diet in mice is considered teratogenic, affecting the function and rate of growth of organs such as brain and heart
> - Serum ketones, calorimetry, and fasting blood sugar should always be monitored whenever a patient is put on diet

be considered as threat, however, it is unclear how it affects fetal metabolism, development, and overall safety.

Some facts about ketosis in healthy and complicated pregnancies are summarized in Box 9.1.

Currently, there is little evidence to recommend any specific diet for optimizing pregnancy outcomes. Outside pregnancy, however, obese women have been tried on low "glycemic index" diets which lead to greater fat loss and better capacity to prevent weight re-gain after a large weight loss. This type of diet and its possible benefit in pregnancy, however, awaits further research before its safe application in pregnancy.

## Use of Prophylactic Metformin

It has been shown that failure of the above-mentioned intervention of dietary and life style modification to improve the outcome of pregnancy complicated by obesity was attributed to patient noncompliance.[80,81] Hence, in the search for an alternative treatment, metformin, an agent, was favorably considered due to its primary role of reducing IR and proven success and safety in the management of gestational diabetes mellitus.[82] Hyperglycemia and increased IR that occur with obesity may explain the association between obesity and fetal macrosomia, as well as other pregnancy complications. Metformin reduces gestational weight gain in GDM patients.[83] Similar effect was noted in obese (BMI > 35) nondiabetic pregnant women who took 3.0 g of metformin from 12 weeks to 18 weeks of gestation until delivery.[84] A randomized double-blinded, placebo-controlled trial on the use of metformin in obese pregnant women, known as the MOP study, which was published recently in the New England Journal of Medicine,[84] had a better design and methodology when compared to the well-known effect of metformin on maternal and fetal outcomes in obese pregnant women (EMPOWaR) study that had shown no significant differences between the metformin group and the placebo group in, maternal gestational weight gain. The MOP study, however, did not confirm any other improvement in perinatal outcome such as the rate of preeclampsia, or the median birth weight.[85] This beneficial effect of metformin was also established in other studies including a Cochrane review protocol.[86]

In addition, metformin has been found to play a major role in reducing inflammatory substances such as IL-6 and CRP. These markers have been associated with adverse outcomes such as PET and premature deliveries in obese pregnant women.[87]

Prenatal metformin administration in animal studies has shown reduced fat mass and better glucose tolerance in adulthood of the offspring born to obese mother.[88] This metformin beneficial effect on future life risk of obesity and metabolic syndrome was demonstrated despite the absence of an effect on birth weight percentile. Similar results were obtained in humans at 2 years of age when children of GDM women who received metformin antenataly had lower visceral body fat.[89]

## INTERVENTION BEFORE PREGNANCY

World Health Organization has reported that around 40% of pregnancies can be unintended; this would diminish the effectiveness of any prepregnancy measures to lose weight unless bariatric surgery was performed. Moreover, significant weight reduction can be achieved before pregnancy with bariatric surgery.

Metabolic surgery, initially designed to promote weight loss (bariatric surgery) have been found recently improving glucose tolerance more effectively than any known pharmaceutical or behavioral approach, relieving many patients from a long-standing disease like type 2 diabetes. The physiological and molecular mechanisms underlying these beneficial glycemic effects remain to be revealed.[90]

Swedish health registries between 2006 and 2011 showed that the risk of GDM and macrosomia were markedly reduced with bariatric surgery when compared to matching group of obese women who did not have bariatric surgery (1.9% vs 6.8%) and (8.6% vs 22.4%), respectively. On the other hand, bariatric surgery was associated with double the risk of delivering small for date babies, while the risk of babies born prematurely was similar between the two groups.[91] Larger RCTs are needed with specific attention to safety and defining a minimum adequate diet for safe maternal weight loss without affecting maternal and fetal health. Long-term effects of weight loss diets during pregnancy without starvation will stipulate future cohorts to monitor the development of degenerative and chronic disease.

## KEY NOTES

- The current findings indicate that prepregnancy counseling and earlier screening and intervention for GDM may result in improved short- and long-term outcomes.
- All obese women should be tested for GDM.
- Although diabetes per se is a much stronger risk factor of PET than BMI, normalization of prepregnancy weight could further reduce the risk of PET in diabetic and nondiabetic women.
- Contrary to the common myth "Eat for two", pregnant women do not need additional food throughout their pregnancy.
- Weight gain in obese women should be limited to 5–9 kg.
- Maternal weight gain during pregnancy is more detrimental on adverse pregnancy outcome than the mothers BMI at the onset of the pregnancy.
- GDM is a preventable disease in young women once obesity is prevented.
- Effective nutrition and physical activity interventions that produce weight loss could prevent type 2 diabetes in obese women who have GDM.

- Metformin can reduce maternal weight gain but does not affect birth weight.
- Metabolic/Bariatric surgery in nonpregnant obese women may improve their future pregnancy outcomes.

## REFERENCES

1. Owens LA, Egan AM, Carmody L, et al. Ten years of optimizing outcomes for women with type 1 and type 2 diabetes in pregnancy—the Atlantic DIP experience. J Clin Endocrinol Metab. 2016;101:1598-605.
2. Chu SY, Callaghan WM, Kim SY, et al. Maternal obesity and risk of gestational diabetes mellitus. Diabetes Care. 2007;30:2070-6.
3. Barquera S, Campos-Nonato I, Hernández-Barrera L, et al. Prevalence of obesity in Mexican adults 2000–2012. Salud Publica Mex. 2013;55(Suppl 2):S151-60.
4. Margaret C Hogan, BianiSaavedra-Avendano, Blair G Darney, et al. Reclassifying causes of obstetric death in Mexico: a repeated cross-sectional study. Bull World Health Organ. 2016;94:362-9.
5. Say L, Chou D, Gemmill A, et al. Global causes of maternal death: a WHO systematic analysis. Lancet Glob Health. 2014;2(6):e323-33.
6. Berrington de Gonzalez A, Hartge P, Cerhan JR, et al. Body-mass index and mortality among 1.46 million white adults. N Engl J Med. 2010;363:2211-9.
7. Obesity: Preventing and Managing the Global Epidemic; World Health Organization (WHO): Geneva, Switzerland, 1998.
8. Rahman M, Berenson AB. Self-perception of weight and its association with weight-related behaviors in young, reproductive-aged women. Obstet Gynecol. 2010;116(6):1274-80.
9. Berenson AB, Pohlmeier AM, Laz TH, et al. Obesity risk knowledge, weight misperception, and diet and health-related attitudes among women intending to become pregnant. J Acad Nutr Diet. 2016;116(1):69-75.
10. Al-Daghri NM, Al-Attas OS, Alokail MS, et al. Diabetes mellitus type 2 and other chronic non-communicable diseases in the central region, Saudi Arabia (riyadh cohort 2): a decade of an epidemic. BMC Med. 2011; 9:76.
11. El-Gilany AH, El-Wehady A. Prevalence of obesity in a Saudi obstetric population. Obes Facts. 2009; 2:217-20.
12. Jang HC. Gestational diabetes in Korea: incidence and risk factors of diabetes in women with previous gestational diabetes. Diabetes Metab J. 2011;35:1-7.
13. Wahabi H, Esmaeil S, Fayed A, et al. Pre-existing diabetes mellitus and adverse pregnancy outcomes. BMC Research Notes. 2012; 5:496.
14. Catalano PM, McIntyre HD, Cruickshank JK, et al. The hyperglycemia and adverse pregnancy outcome study: associations of GDM and obesity with pregnancy outcomes. Diabetes Care. 2012;35:780-6.
15. Ricart W, Lopez J, Mozas J, et al. Body mass index has a greater impact on pregnancy outcomes than gestational hyperglycaemia. Diabetologia. 2005;48:1736-42.
16. Wahabi HA, Fayed AA, Alzeidan RA, et al. The independent effects of maternal obesity and gestational diabetes on pregnancy outcomes. BMC Endocrine Disorder. 2014;14:47.
17. Athukorala C, Rumbold AR, Willson KJ, et al. The risk of adverse pregnancy outcomes in women who are overweight or obese. BMC Pregnancy Childbirth. 2010;10:56.
18. Crowther CA, Hiller JE, Moss JR, et al. Effect of treatment of gestational diabetes mellitus on pregnancy outcomes. N Engl J Med. 2005;352:2477-86.
19. Gillman MW, Rifas-Shiman S, Berkey CS, et al. Maternal gestational diabetes, birth weight, and adolescent obesity. Pediatrics. 2003;111:e221-e226.
20. Fetal Macrosomia. Report no. 22. Washington, DC, The American College of Obstetricians and Gynecologists, 2000.

21. Jolly MC, Sebire NJ, Harris JP, et al. Risk factors for macrosomia and its clinical consequences: a study of 350,311 pregnancies. Eur J Obstet Gynecol Reprod Biol. 2003;111:9-14.
22. Rasmussen SA, Chu SY, Kim SY, et al. Maternal obesity and risk of neural tube defects: a meta-analysis. Am J Obstet Gynecol. 2008;198(6):611-9.
23. Mojtabai R. Body mass index and serum folate in childbearing age women. Eur J Epidemiol. 2004;19(11):1029.
24. Pedersen J. Diabetes and pregnancy; blood sugar of newborn infants during fasting and glucose administration. Ugeskr Laeger. 1952;114:685.
25. Schwartz R, Gruppuso PA, Petzold K, et al. Hyperinsulinemia and macrosomia in the fetus of the diabetic mother. Diabetes Care. 1994;17:640-8.
26. Griffiths LJ, Dezateux C, Cole TJ. Differential parental weight and height contributions to offspring birthweight and weight gain in infancy. Int J Epidemiol. 2007;36:104-7.
27. Ramsay JE, Ferrell WR, Crawford L, et al. Maternal obesity is associated with dysregulation of metabolic, vascular, and inflammatory pathways. J Clin Endocrinol Metab. 2002;87:4231-7.
28. Schaefer-Graf UM, Graf K, Kulbacka I, et al. Maternal lipids as strong determinants of fetal environment and growth in pregnancies with gestational diabetes mellitus. Diabetes Care. 2008;31:1858-63.
29. Retnakaran R, Ye C, Hanley AJ, et al. Effect of maternal weight, adipokines, glucose intolerance and lipids on infant birth weight among women without gestational diabetes mellitus. CMAJ. 2012;184:1353-60.
30. Evers IM, de Valk HW, Mol BW, et al. Macrosomia despite good glycaemic control in Type I diabetic pregnancy; results of a nationwide study in The Netherlands. Diabetologia. 2002;45:1484-9.
31. Sovio U, Murphy HR, Smith GC. Accelerated fetal growth prior to diagnosis of GDM: a prospective cohort study of nulliparous women. Diabetes Care. 2016.
32. Chu SY, Kim SY, Schmid CH, et al. Maternal obesity and risk of cesarean delivery: a meta-analysis. Obes Rev. 2007;8:385-94.
33. Dietz PM, Callaghan WM, Morrow B, et al. Population-based assessment of the risk of primary cesarean delivery due to excess prepregnancy weight among nulliparous women delivering term infants. Matern Child Health J. 2005;9:237-44.
34. Young TK, Woodmansee B. Factors that are associated with cesarean delivery in a large private practice: the importance of prepregnancy body mass index and weight gain. Am J Obstet Gynecol. 2002;187:312-8.
35. Vahratian A, Zhang J, Troendle JF, et al. Maternal prepregnancy overweight and obesity and the pattern of labor progression in term nulliparous women. Obstet Gynecol. 2004;104:943-51.
36. Cnattingius R, Cnattingius S, Notzon FC. Obstacles to reducing cesarean rates in a low-cesarean setting: the effect of maternal age, height, and weight. Obstet Gynecol. 1998;92:501-6.
37. Sebire NJ, Jolly M, Harris JP, et al. Maternal obesity and pregnancy outcome: a study of 287,213 pregnancies in London. Int J Obes Relat Metab Disord. 2001;25:1175-82.
38. Tomoda S, Tamura T, Sudo Y, et al. Effects of obesity on pregnant women: maternal hemodynamic change. Am J Perinatol. 1996;13:73-8.
39. Edwards LE, Hellerstedt WL, Alton IR, et al. Pregnancy complications and birth outcomes in obese and normal weight women: effects of gestational weight change. Obstet Gynecol. 1996;87:389-94.
40. Ijuin H, Douchi T, Nakamura S, et al. Possible association of body-fat distribution with preeclampsia. J Obstet Gynaecol Res. 1997;23:45-9.
41. Hyperglycemia and Adverse Pregnancy Outcome (HAPO) Study Cooperative Research Group. Hyperglycemia and Adverse Pregnancy Outcome (HAPO) study: preeclampsia. Am J Obstet Gynecol. 2010;202(255):e251–e257.
42. Sohlberg S, Stephansson O, Cnattingius S, et al. Maternal body mass index, height, and risks of preeclampsia. Am J Hypertens. 2012;25:120-5.

43. Jarvie E, Hauguel-de-Mouzon S, Nelson SM, et al. Lipotoxicity in obese pregnancy and its potential role in adverse pregnancy outcome and obesity in the offspring. Clin Sci (Lond). 2010;119: 123-9.

44. Harmon AC, Cornelius DC, Amaral LM, et al. The role of inflammation in the pathology of preeclampsia. Clin Sci. 2016;130:409-19.

45. Roberts JM, Bodnar LM, Patrick TE, et al. The role of obesity in preeclampsia. Pregnancy Hypertens. 2011;1:6-16.

46. Persson M, Pasupathy D, Hanson U, et al. Pre-pregnancy body mass index and the risk of adverse outcome in type 1 diabetic pregnancies: a population-based cohort study. BMJ Open. 2012;2:e000601.

47. Cundy T, Slee F, Gamble G, et al. Hypertensive disorders of pregnancy in women with Type 1 and Type 2 diabetes. Diabet Med: J Br Diabet Assoc. 2002;19:482-9.

48. Balsells M, Garcia-Patterson A, Gich I, et al. Maternal and fetal outcome in women with type 2 versus type 1 diabetes mellitus: a systematic review and metaanalysis. J Clin Endocrinol Metab. 2009;94:4284-91.

49. Persson M, Cnattingius S, Wikstrom AK, et al. Maternal overweight and obesity and risk of preeclampsia in women with type 1 diabetes or type 2 diabetes. Diabetologia. 2016;59: 2099-105.

50. Starikov R, Inman K, Chen K, et al. Comparison of placental findings in type 1 and type 2 diabetic pregnancies. Placenta. 2014;35:1001-6.

51. Damm JA, Asbjornsdottir B, Callesen NF, et al. Diabetic nephropathy and microalbuminuria in pregnant women with type 1 and type 2 diabetes: prevalence, antihypertensive strategy, and pregnancy outcome. Diabetes Care. 2013;36:3489-94.

52. Landon MB. Diabetic nephropathy and pregnancy. Clin Obstet Gynecol 2007;50:998-1006.

53. Klemetti MM, Laivuori H, Tikkanen M, et al. Obstetric and perinatal outcome in type 1 diabetes patients with diabetic nephropathy during 1988–2011. Diabetologia. 2015;58:678-86.

54. Yogev Y, Chen R, Ben-Haroush A, et al. Maternal overweight and pregnancy outcome in women with Type-1 diabetes mellitus and different degrees of nephropathy. J Matern Fetal Neonatal Med: Off J Eur Assoc Perinat Med Fed Asia Oceania Perinat Soc Int Soc Perinat Obstet. 2010;23: 999-1003.

55. Jensen DM, Damm P, Ovesen P, et al. Microalbuminuria, preeclampsia, and preterm delivery in pregnant women with type 1 diabetes: results from a nationwide Danish study. Diabetes Care. 2010;33:90-4.

56. Hiilesmaa V, Suhonen L, Teramo K. Glycaemic control is associated with pre-eclampsia but not with pregnancy-induced hypertension in women with type I diabetes mellitus. Diabetologia. 2000;43:1534-9.

57. Duckitt K, Harrington D. Risk factors for pre-eclampsia at antental booking: systemic review of controlled studies. Br Med J (Clin Res Ed). 2005;330:549-50.

58. Gordin D, Forsblom C, Groop PH, et al. Risk factors of hypertensive pregnancies in women with diabetes and the influence on their future life. Ann Med. 2014;46:498-502.

59. Confidential Enquiry into Maternal and Child Health. Perinatal mortality 2005: England, Wales and Northern Ireland. London: CEMACH; 2007.

60. Tennant PW, Rankin J, Bell R. Maternal body mass index and the risk of fetal and infant death: a cohort study from the North of England. Hum Reprod. 2011;26(6):1501-11.

61. Meehan S, Beck CR, Mair-Jenkins J, et al. Maternal obesity and infant mortality: a meta-analysis. Pediatrics. 2014;133(5):863-71.

62. Johansson S, Villamor E, Altman M, et al. Maternal overweight and obesity in early pregnancy and risk of infant mortality: a population based cohort study in Sweden, 2014.

63. Aune D, Saugstad O, Henriksen T, et al. Maternal body mass index and the risk of fetal death, stillbirth, and infant death: a systematic review and meta-analysis. JAMA. 2014;311(15): 1536-46.

64. Homan GF, Davies M, Norman R. The impact of lifestyle factors on reproductive performance in the general population and those undergoing infertility treatment: a review. Hum Reprod Update. 2007;13(3):209-23.

65. Shaw GM, Wise PH, Mayo J, et al. Maternal prepregnancy body mass index and risk of spontaneous preterm birth. Pediatr Perinat Epidemiol. 2014;28:302-11.

66. Van den Akker CH, Schierbeek H, Dorst KY, et al. Human fetal amino acid metabolism at term gestation. Am J Clin Nutr. 2009;89:153-60.

67. Felig P, Kim YJ, Lynch V, et al. Amino acid metabolism during starvation in human pregnancy. J Clin Invest. 1972;51:1195-202.

68. Frise CJ, Mackillop L, Joash K, et al. Starvation ketoacidosis in pregnancy. Eur J Obstet Gynecol Reprod Biol. 2013;167:1-7.

69. Metzger BE, Ravnikar V, Vileisis RA, et al. Accelerated starvation and the skipped breakfast in late normal pregnancy. Lancet. 1982;1:588-92.

70. Khoshdel A, Kheiri S, Hashemi-Dehkordi E, et al. The effect of Ramadan fasting on LH, FSH, oestrogen, progesterone and leptin in pregnant women. J Obstet Gynaecol. 2014;34:634-8.

71. Ziaee V, Kihanidoost Z, Younesian M, et al. The effect of ramadan fasting on outcome of pregnancy. Iran J Pediatr. 2010;20:181-6.

72. Herrmann TS, Siega-Riz AM, Hobel CJ, et al. Prolonged periods without food intake during pregnancy increase risk for elevated maternal corticotropin-releasing hormone concentrations. Am J Obstet Gynecol. 2001;185:403-12.

73. Oken E, Kleinman KP, Belfort MB, et al. Associations of gestational weight gain with short and longer-term maternal and child health outcomes. Am J Epidemiol. 2009;170:173-80.

74. Kershaw EE, Flier JS. Adipose tissue as an endocrine organ. J Clin Endocrinol Metab. 2004;89:2548-56.

75. Catalano PM. Obesity, insulin resistance, and pregnancy outcome. Reproduction. 2010;140:365-71.

76. Butte NF. Carbohydrate and lipid metabolism in pregnancy: Normal compared with gestational diabetes mellitus. Am J Clin Nutr. 2000;71:1256S-1261S.

77. Van den Akker CH, Schierbeek H, Dorst KY, et al. Human fetal amino acid metabolism at term gestation. Am J Clin Nutr. 2009;89:153-60.

78. Magee MS, Knopp RH, Benedetti TJ. Metabolic effects of 1200-kcal diet in obese pregnant women with gestational diabetes. Diabetes. 1990;39:234-40.

79. Sussman D, van Eede M, Wong MD, et al. Effects of a ketogenic diet during pregnancy on embryonic growth in the mouse. BMC Pregnancy and Childbirth. 2013;13:109.

80. Rogozinska E, Chamillard M, Hitman GA, et al. Nutritional manipulation for the primary prevention of gestational diabetes mellitus: a meta-analysis of randomised studies. PLoS One. 2015;10(2):e0115526.

81. Poston L, Bell R, Croker H, et al. Effect of a behavioural intervention in obese pregnant women (the UPBEAT study): a multi-centre, randomised controlled trial. Lancet Diabetes Endocrinol. 2015;3:767-77.

82. Cassina M, Donà M, Di Gianantonio E, et al. First-trimester exposure to metformin and risk of birth defects: a systematic review and meta-analysis. Hum Reprod Update. 2014;20:656-69.

83. Balani J, Hyer SL, Rodin DA, et al. Pregnancy outcomes in women with gestational diabetes treated with metformin or insulin: a case-control study. Diabet Med. 2009;26:798-802.

84. Syngelaji A, Nicolaides KH, Balani J, et al. Metformin versus placebo in obese pregnant women without diabetes mellitus. N Engl J Med. 2016;374:434-43.

85. Chiswick C, Reynolds RM, Denison F, et al. Effect of metformin on maternal and fetal outcomes in obese pregnant women (EMPOWaR): a randomized, double-blind, placebo-controlled trial. Lancet Diabetes Endocrinol. 2015;3:778-86.

86. Eames AJ, Grivell RM, Deussen AR, et al. Metformin for women who are obese during pregnancy for improving maternal and infant outcomes. Cochrane Database Syst Rev. 2013;6:CD010564.

87. Xu L, Lee M, Jeyabalan A, et al. The relationship of hypovitaminosis D and IL-6 in preeclampsia. Am J Obstet Gynecol. 2014;210:149 e1-7.

88. Alomaki H, Heinaniemi M, Vahatalo LH, et al. Prenatal metformin exposure in a maternal high fat diet mouse model alters the transcriptome and modifies the metabolic responses of the offspring. PLoS One. 2014;9:e115778.

89. Rowan JA, Hague WM, Gao W, et al. Metformin versus insulin for the treatment of gestational diabetes. N Engl J Med. 2008;358:2003-15.

90. Cefalu WT, Rubino F, Cummings DE. Metabolic surgery for type 2 diabetes: changing the landscape of diabetes care. Diabetes Care. 2016;39(6):857-60.

91. Johansson K, Cnattingius S, Näslund I, et al. Outcomes of pregnancy after bariatric surgery. N Engl J Med. 2015;372:814-24.

# Index

Page numbers followed by *b* refer to box, *f* refer to figure, and *t* refer to table.